The Psychoses of Epilepsy

The Psychoses of Epilepsy

Michael R. Trimble, F.R.C.P., F.R.C.PSYCH.

Consultant Physician
Department of Psychological Medicine
The National Hospitals
Queen Square, London

Raymond-Way Reader in Behavioural Neurology
Department of Neurology,
Institute of Neurology
Queen Square, London

Raven Press 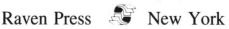 New York

Raven Press, Ltd., 1185 Avenue of the Americas, New York, New York 10036

Made in the United States of America

Library of Congress Cataloging-in-Publication Data

Trimble, Michael R.
    The psychoses of epilepsy / by Michael R. Trimble.
       p.   cm.
    Includes bibliographical references.
    Includes index.
    ISBN 0-88167-739-6
    1. Epilepsy—Complications and sequelae. 2. Psychoses.
  I. Title.
    [DNLM: 1. Epilepsy—psychology. 2. Psychotic Disorders. WL 385
T831p]
RC372.T73 1991
616.8′53—dc20
DNLM/DLC
for Library of Congress   90-9045
                                                CIP

9 8 7 6 5 4 3 2 1

To Mary Raymond-Way

Preface

In recent years the subject of the psychoses of epilepsy has occasioned much controversy. In some ways this is surprising. Brief review of the literature reveals that patients with psychosis and epilepsy (described in various ways, dependent upon the historical time and culture), have been reported since the earliest of medical writings. In some cultures, historically, the words used for epilepsy and psychosis were intertwined. For example, in Japan, epilepsy is referred to as *ten-kan*. However, the term *tenkyo* was also popularly used, *ten* referring to epilepsy, and *kyo* referring to psychosis (Akimoto, 1982). Similarly, in Chinese medicine, *dian* refers both to epilepsy and insanity and is sometimes put with *k'uang* or *Feng* (mania or psychosis) to form the compound words *dian k'uang* or *feng-dang* (Lai and Lai 1990). Even within our own language, the term *lunatic* implies a sudden movement disorder within the setting of madness.

In support of these historical connections, anyone charged with the care of many patients with epilepsy will, upon careful observation, witness episodes of psychosis, either in the ictal phase or the postictal phase of the illness. Regardless of these associations, resistance to an acceptance of any form of association between epilepsy and psychiatric illness, let alone psychosis, is a viewpoint commonly encountered. There are several obvious reasons for this. First, epilepsy is one clinical diagnosis while, for example, schizophrenia is another with very different features. At first sight, rejection of an association is simple. Second, to propose that patients with periodic psychiatric states have ictal or epileptic "equivalents" is not only unscientific, it would seem unnecessary. Patients either have epilepsy or they do not. Finally, it is considered an injustice to many people with epilepsy to confuse and muddle up psychiatry with epilepsy. It may stigmatise one at the expense of the other, and may opacify concepts which seem so clear: for example, what is epilepsy?

Whatever the arguments, there is much literature on the subject, most of which has not been collated before. It is the purpose of this monograph to explore and evaluate the association. Some of the conclusions reached may not wholly satisfy all readers. They are, however, in keeping with thinking in the biological neurosciences generally, in particular in the arena of neuropsychiatry.

In part the review is to explore a body of literature, most of which is not widely known, even to scholars interested in the links or absence of links between psychoses and epilepsy. The majority of the literature since the middle of the last century has been covered, and of necessity an historical approach has been taken to interpretation.

Chapter One explores the history of the relationship between epilepsy and psychosis, bringing us up to the middle of this century. Many of the arguments found here are rehearsed again in the modern era, which may be said to have begun in the 1940s and 1950s. This related to the pioneering work of such investigators as Gibbs in the United States, Hill and Pond in the United Kingdom, and Gastaut in France. All were exploring the clinical use of the newly introduced electroencephalogram in clinical practise, and made observations on associations between temporal lobe abnormalities and ensuing psychopathology.

Classification is of great importance in clinical practice, and has bearing on the subject of the interictal psychoses described in later chapters. Chapters Two and Three thus concentrate on issues of classification in epilepsy and in psychiatry, especially with regard to personality disorders and psychoses. It is hoped that these will be of interest to neurologists wishing to understand more about psychiatric taxonomy and to psychiatrists who wish to be better versed on more recent ways of classifying seizure disorders.

Chapter Four is a brief excursion into neuroanatomy, neurochemistry, and neuropathology with special relevance for epilepsy. The importance of understanding the essential elements and hodology of the limbic system and its functions are stressed.

The literature on the psychoses of epilepsy comprises the remaining chapters of the book. Chapter Five is devoted to ictal and peri-ictal mental states that are either frankly psychotic or have relevance for an understanding of the psychoses. In Chapter Six the interesting phenomenon of forced normalisation is reviewed. The concern of Chapter Seven is postoperative psychoses, especially following temporal lobectomy. In this chapter the possibility that psychoses develop *de novo* following temporal lobectomy in some patients is raised.

Chapters Eight and Nine review the extensive literature on the interictal psychoses of epilepsy, mainly in relationship to schizophrenia-like states, but also the smaller literature on affective disorders. Risk factors are highlighted, as are phenomenological issues.

Chapter Ten is a clinical review of treatments that are available for the management of epilepsy and for psychoses, with some basic guidelines as to the use of anticonvulsants in patients with psychotic conditions, and the psychopharmacology of the management of psychotic conditions in epilepsy.

The final chapter is an attempt to synthesise the reviewed work on the psychoses of epilepsy. Associations between seizures, psychoses, temporal lobe abnormalities, and psychotic states, especially those presenting with symptoms of schizophrenia, are brought together. It is suggested that an understanding of the psychoses of epilepsy forms an important link between neurology and psychiatry, especially in attempting to clarify certain brain behaviour relationships.

This book should be of interest to academic neurologists and psychiatrists alike, and to all professionals who treat, manage, or encounter, at many levels, patients with epilepsy.

Michael R. Trimble

Acknowledgments

The author is grateful to Dr. Hartmut Meierkord for translations of certain German texts into English, and to Dr. Ley Sander for his preparation of Figure 5.1.

The author is also grateful to many colleagues with whom he has discussed the difficult subject of the psychoses of epilepsy over many stimulating hours.

Contents

The Psychoses of Epilepsy

That epilepsie is sometimes cured by the help of medicines, experience doth testifie. . . . in the meantime, as to what further belongs to the prognostication of this disease, if it end not about the time of ripe age, neither can be driven away by the use of remedies, there happens a diverse event in several sick patients, for it either ends immediately in death, or is changed into some other disease, to wit, the palsie, stupiditie, or melancholy, for the most part incurable.

Willis, 1667

1

Historical Introduction

The history of epilepsy is closely associated with that of psychiatry. Both have links with gods, demons, witches, and the supernatural; and have evoked prejudice, disaffection, and malediction from other members of society. Reference to psychiatric illness and epilepsy can be found in the earliest of medical writings; but further, their symbiotic relationship has been a persistent historical theme.

It is widely acknowledged that the disease the Greeks called "sacred" referred to epilepsy, and the first monograph on the subject was that of Hippocrates (460–377 BC). "On the Sacred Disease" was a medical text written largely for lay readers, and its central theme was that epilepsy was not sacred or divine, but a natural affection with an hereditary origin. The Greeks, it seems, surmised that epilepsy was divine because it was wonderful: only a God could throw a man to the ground, convulse him, and then restore him to normality.

Hippocrates noted that it did not affect all men equally, attacking the phlegmatic and not the bilious. This was associated with its pathogenesis which was due to disease of the brain. However, Hippocrates also pronounced: "Men ought to know that from nothing else but thence [from the brain] comes joys, delights, laughter and sports, and sorrows griefs, despondency, and lamentations . . . and by this same organ we become mad and delirious, and fears and terrors assail us. . . . As long as the brain is at rest, the man enjoys his reason, but the depravement of the brain arises from phlegm and bile" (1939, p. 366).

The brain was thus the seat of both the falling sickness and madness, and both were related to phlegm.

There are early examples of the association of the sacred disease to madness. Herodotus, discussing the mad behaviour of the Persian king Cambyses, says that from birth he suffered from "a certain great disease . . . which some people call sacred. And thus it would not be unlikely that if the body suffered from a great disease the mind was not sound either" (Temkin, 1971, p. 15).

Hippocrates himself mused on the lay notions of the disease, stating that "terrors which happen during the night, and fevers, and delirium, and jumpings out of bed, and frightful apparitions, and fleeing away,—all these they hold to be plots of Hecate, and the invasions of the Heroes" (p. 358).

Hecate was the moon goddess, sometimes merged with Artemis, to whom was attributed, amongst other things, raving and madness.

Hercules, whose birth was delayed by Hera to favour the earlier delivery and hence succession of Eurystheus to the title of ruler of Greece, may have had epilepsy, and is said to have killed his own children in a seizure of madness. The supposition that this was epileptic relates to a comment in a Hippocratic treatise that "when the uterus is near the liver and the hypochondrium and produces suffocation, the woman turns up the white of her eyes, becomes cold, gnashes her teeth, saliva flows into her mouth, and she resembles the persons seized by the Herculean disease" (Temkin, p. 20).

Although this does not definitively state that Hippocrates was referring to epilepsy, it is suggestive. This quote also serves to illustrate another historical link between epilepsy and psychiatry; namely, that between hysteria and epilepsy (Trimble, 1981, 1989).

Further evidence comes from the writings of Aristotle. In considering the question of why talented individuals are always melancholic, he gives Hercules as an example: "For he apparently had this constitution and therefore epileptic afflictions were called after him 'the sacred disease' by the ancients. His mad fit in the incident with the children points to this" (Simon, 1978, p. 229).

In the Euripides version, Hercules falls to the ground, sleeps, and is then amnesic for the whole event.

The association between epilepsy and melancholy is another theme of the Greek and Roman physicians. Hippocrates stated: "Melancholics ordinarily become epileptics, and epileptics melancholics: of these two states, what determines the preference is the direction the malady takes; if it bears upon the body, epilepsy, if upon the intelligence, melancholy" (Lewis, 1934).

Aretaeus noted that people with epilepsy were "languid, spiritless . . . unsociable, and not disposed to hold intercourse, nor to be sociable, at any period of life; sleepless, subject to many horrid dreams, and without appetite" (Adams, 1856).

These ideas link with the Galenic concept of humours and their relationship to temperament. The latter was construed as a somatic rather than a psychological state, and was derived by combination of four basic humours: phlegm, blood, black bile, and yellow bile. The melancholic disposition was related to black bile, but it was also related to "raving," and to epilepsy. For Galen, the two had a related pathogenesis: "This humour arises in some people in large quantity either because of their original humoural constitution or by their customary diet which is transformed into this humour by digestion in the blood vessels. Like thick phlegm, this heavy atrabilious blood obstructs the passage through the middle or posterior cavity of the brain and sometimes causes epilepsy. When its excess pervades the brain matter itself, it causes melancholy" (Siegel, 1973).

LUNATICS

There is a clear association in historical writings between the moon, epilepsy, and insanity. The Gospels provide an early example. The ninth chapter of the Gospel of

Mark (9:17–22, 26–27) with additions in italics from Matthew's and Luke's versions of the same incident, reads as follows:

> Master, I have brought to thee my son *for he is a lunatic and sore vexed* [and] hath a dumb spirit; and wheresoever he taketh him, he teareth him: *and bruising him hardly departeth from him*; and he foameth and gnasheth with his teeth, and pineth away. . . .
> And they brought him unto Him: and when He saw him straightway the spirit tare him; and he fell on the ground, and wallowed foaming. And He asked his father, How long is it ago since this came unto him? And he said, Of a child. And ofttimes it hath cast him into the fire and into the water to destroy him: *And Jesus rebuked the unclean spirit, and he departed out of him*. . . . and he was as one dead . . . but Jesus took him by the hand, and lifted him up; and he arose.

In Rome epilepsy was known as *morbidus lunaticus*. Aretaeus referred to it as an affliction of persons who have sinned against the moon, and it was a widely held belief that the timing of seizures was related to the light of the moon, with a tendency to have attacks at full moon. The term *lunatic* thus embraced periodic affections, including epilepsy, but also varieties of mental illness. The astrologist Julius Firmicius Maternus, in the fourth century AD, noted that the moon made people convulsed or lunatic, and referred to *lunaticos epilempticos* (Temkin, p. 94).

MIDDLE AGES

With the waning of Greek influence on Roman scholars, few advancements in medical thinking emerged until the Renaissance. The centre of learning moved to the Arab world, and few new ideas on epilepsy emerged. The great Rhazes (AD 865–925) believed in lunar theories; the associations between demons, madness, and epilepsy remained. The writer Ali b. Rabban al-Tabari referred to epilepsy as "the diviner's disease," emphasising the prophetic powers of some epileptics (Temkin, 1971). Although the relationship between religiosity and epilepsy is referred to later, the visions of many soothsayers and prophets have been suggested as manifestations of epilepsy.

A good example from this era is Mohammed (AD 570–623). Born in Mecca, his possible epilepsy seems to have been denied by the Islamic tradition and promulgated largely by Christian writers. He is reported to have had attacks in which he became pale, resembled a drunkard, fell down, and sweated profusely. At such times he had visual and auditory hallucinations. After several years of such attacks, in which the angel Gabriel came before him, he came to see himself as a prophet. Nonetheless, the inhabitants of Mecca considered him to be a madman and one possessed, and his wife thought he was a fanatic deceived by the artifices of a demon (Howden, 1873).

A Christian equivalent was Saint Paul of Tarsus (Landsborough, 1987). He, too, had ecstatic visions, was spurned by the Galatians because of some illness, and certainly during his conversion he "dropped to the ground and heard a voice" (Acts 9:18).

Thus Mohammed and Saint Paul were possible examples of people with epilepsy who had episodes which would today be referred to as psychotic, but with associated religiosity. There is a considerable amount of ancient literature emphasising the associations between epilepsy, ecstasy, and prophecy (Temkin, 1971), themes which are continually revived up to the present day (see p. 128).

More specific associations of epilepsy and insanity are hard to find in the Middle Ages. Benivieni described automatic behaviour, and early accounts of what are now referred to as partial seizures are recorded. Such observations allowed Marci (1595–1667) to broaden the definition of epilepsy to "any affection of the body where the victims are disordered in their minds, while the members (of the body), be it all, or some, are moved against their will" (Temkin, 1971, p. 192).

Shakespeare, however, may have had insights:

Iago.   My Lord is fall'n into an epilepsy:
            This is his second fit; he had one yesterday.
Cassio.   Rub him about the temples.
Iago.   No, forbear;
            The lethargy must have his quiet course:
            If not, he foams at mouth; and by and by
            Breaks out to savage madness. . . .
                            (*Othello IV,i,51–57*)

THE EIGHTEENTH CENTURY

With the enlightenment came attempts to oppose supernatural and demonic explanations for disease, but epilepsy was bound by its historical association with possession. This extended far beyond lay and theological considerations and was reflected in the writings of such physicians as Stahl (1695–1734), Hoffmann (1660–1742), van Swieten (1700–1772) and even Willis (1621–1675). In 1729 an English doctor, Harle, wrote: "Tis true, in one place a person is said to have a devil, and be mad, and another to be demoniack, and yet is called a lunatic, or one troubled with the falling sickness. If we take in both texts, we have the full meaning, which is, that the madness and epilepsy these people labour'd under were caus'd by the devil" (Harle, 1729, p. 22).

The influence of the moon was still in evidence. Richard Mead (1673–1754), in his "Treatise Concerning the Influence of the Sun and Moon upon Human Bodies, and the Diseases thereby produced," wrote that epileptic fits "do constantly recur every new and full moon . . . the Latins [called sufferers] . . . Lunatici . . . and it may not be improper to remark in this place, that the raving fits of mad people, which keep lunar periods, are generally accompanied with epileptic symptoms: which was attested to me as a constant observation by the late learned Dr. Tyson, formerly physician to Bethlem Hospital, who upon that account usually called such patients epileptic mad" (Mead, 1746).

The first substantial treatise on epilepsy was that published by Tissot (1728–1797) in 1770. Although opposing the ideas of lunar influences, he introduced another obliquity; namely, an association between masturbation and epilepsy. His book *L'onanism* (Tissot, 1782) spelled out the consequences of masturbation, which included epilepsy, venereal pleasures in general being one cause of sympathetic epilepsy (Tissot, 1770). His ideas influenced thinking on epilepsy for over a hundred years, and were related to the later introduction of bromides for treatment. Likewise, the idea that masturbation caused insanity lived on for several generations.

THE NINETEENTH CENTURY

The growth of the hospital system led to concentrations of patients with various problems coming under close medical scrutiny. Many patients with epilepsy previously incarcerated in prisons along with the insane were now to be found in hospital wards, the progression of their illnesses, if chronic, being observed and documented. Epilepsy was a particularly prominent diagnosis in the asylums, and in some, epileptic patients were segregated into separate wards. The Commissioners in Lunacy reported that in 1887 there were 1,294 patients with epilepsy in various asylums in England and Wales, from a total of 14,336; and 9% of insane patients brought under treatment that year had epilepsy (Savage, 1892).

Older asylums, for example: Bethlem, Bethel Hospital, Norwich, and Saint Luke's, excluded patients with epilepsy from admission. Griesinger (1857) recorded that the prognosis for epilepsy associated with insanity was so bad that asylums that were devoted to curable cases of insanity "shut their gates against all insane persons . . . affected with epilepsy" (Griesinger, p. 406).

Later-built, new county asylums, however, did admit epileptic patients, and for the first time the prognosis of the disease could be studied. One consequence was that asylum physicians saw severe cases, less affected patients staying under the care of general physicians and, later, neurologists.

Pinel (1745–1826), one of the leading physicians in Paris, was physician in chief at the Bicêtre and at the Salpêtrière. He is credited, along with William Tuke (1732–1822) and Connolly (1794–1866), with the so-called unchaining of patients in the then asylum-workhouses in which they were incarcerated. He recognised "insanity complicated with epilepsy," which he noted was frequent in the hospital setting and was incurable. Interestingly, he advocated separation of epileptic patients from others:

> Few objects are found to inspire so much horror and repugnance amongst maniacs in general, than the sight of epileptic fits. . . . Hence it ought to be a fundamental law in all lunatic asylums, to insulate epileptics with great care, and to apportion for their exclusive use part of the establishment, which cannot be visited or seen into by the other classes of lunatics.

He later continued:

> The duties of the superintendent, in respect to this class of maniacs, consists in guarding them against falls and bruises, obviating all causes of strong or intense emotions, preventing errors in regimen or diet, and prescribing exercises suitable to their inclinations and capacities. (1962, pp. 204–205)

Esquirol (1772–1840), one of Pinel's pupils, also recognised insanity associated with epilepsy and its incurable nature. He echoed his master's words that epileptic patients should be separated since: "la vue d'un accès d'épilepsie suffit pour rendre épileptique une personne bien portante. Combien plus grande est le danger pour un aliéné quelquefois si impressionnable" (Esquirol, 1845, p. 331).

Esquirol made a special study of the association between epilepsy and psychiatric illness. He reported that of 339 women at the Salpêtrière with epilepsy, 12 were monomaniacs, 36 were manics, 34 were furious, and 145 were in a state of dementia.

Bouchet and Cazauvieilh (1825) presented pathological data on patients with epilepsy, epilepsy and insanity, and insanity without epilepsy. Similar lesions were noted in all three groups, and they had several cases of epilepsy and insanity with pathology in the Cornes d'Ammon. They concluded that insanity was related to alterations of gray matter and epilepsy to change in white matter. Both were related to congestion and chronic inflammation.

Two other French physicians made a special study of the psychiatric aspects of epilepsy, namely, Morel (1809–1879) and Falret (1824–1902). Falret, a student of Esquirol, introduced a classification of the mental disorders associated with epilepsy that has had a lasting usefulness. Thus he recognised peri-ictal disorders, those associated in time with the seizure; those that were inter-paroxysmal; and patients who entered a prolonged delirium, *folie épileptique*, epileptic insanity proper (Falret 1860, 1861).

Morel seems to have been responsible for the initial concept of the epileptic character. He noted: "Il est dans la nature des maladies nerveuses d'imprimer à l'idiosyncrasie physique et morale des malades un cachet tout à fait particulier" (Reynolds, 1861).

Included were anger, irritability, and fury, and from these ideas grew the concept of *epilepsie larvée*—so-called larval or masked epilepsy. Morel recognised that paroxysmal behaviour disturbances could coincide with the ictus or be independent of it. It was a short step, therefore, to suggesting the concept of epilepsy without seizures, masked and identified by behavioural features only. Morel gave a list of these, discussed in more detail by Berrios (1979). They included marked instability of character, increased motor activity, polymorphic delusions, sudden explosive behaviour, episodic repetition of stereotyped insanity, and sudden shouting. These were elements derived from his description of the epileptic character.

This idea received support from the writings of Falret. Under his third category, *folie épileptique*, he recognised cases in which the slight epileptic paroxysms went unrecognised, or may develop later in the course of the illness. However, he also noted that in some cases, "le délire épileptique se substitue en quelque sorte aux convulsions épileptiques." The convulsions and the delirium were thus both manifestations of the same underlying pathology. Falret further divided epileptic insanity into two forms, namely, *petit mal* and *grand mal intellectuel*. The former were generally milder, although he recognised that in many cases the form was intermediate. The automatism, a subject not new to forensic medicine at that time, was a manifestation of the lesser attacks, and Falret stressed that during them there was a propensity for irrational and violent acts to be carried out.

These views did not receive universal approbation. Herpin (1799–1865), who wrote a major text on epilepsy, published in 1857, in which prognosis was carefully considered, scarcely mentions psychiatric problems. Similarly, in England, several authors were sceptical. Reynolds actually produced statistics on his own patients. He concluded that "epilepsy does not necessarily involve any mental change" (Reynolds, 1861, p. 46), and that while depression of spirits and excitability of temper were common, "ulterior mental changes are rare." Unfortunately, this view is biased since, as he noted, his statistics were on a group in which he excluded all cases of "positive insanity."

Sieveking (1861) explained the dilemma, still echoed in criticisms today:

> There is some difficulty in obtaining satisfactory statistics on this point (insanity in epilepsy). . . . because confirmed epileptics are so frequently removed from the observation of the physician who saw the commencement of the disease, to be placed in asylums; hence the statistics of these establishments only refer to a certain proportion, but by no means all epileptics, as they exclude nearly all cases that have been cured, or in whom the disease has not reached a maximum intensity (Sieveking, 1861, p. 78).

He went on to quote the figures given by Esquirol.

The most important English writer on epilepsy in the last century was Hughlings Jackson (1835–1911). He had much to say on the relationship between epilepsy and mental disorders, and his philosophy of cerebral function and how it was affected in disease embraced four main tenets. These were: the evolution of nervous functions, the hierarchy of those functions, the negative and positive symptoms of dissolution, and the distinction between local and uniform dissolution. The brain was seen as developing in both space and time and was not the static organ of the pathological laboratory. Further, it was hierarchically organised, not a simple collection of reflexes. With any lesion there are two effects: one due to the destruction of tissue, resulting in negative symptoms; the other due to release of subjacent activity of other healthy areas of brain, causing positive symptoms.

Writing as a physician whose territory was the wards of the newly established National Hospital for the Paralysed and Epileptic, Hughlings Jackson saw patients with self-limited episodes of mental change. He advocated that the study of mental diseases could well begin in such a setting. He quoted with approval the figure of Bucknill and Tuke that 6% of patients in asylums "owe their insanity to epilepsy" (Taylor, 1958, p. 119). He felt that cases in which the manifestations of the epilepsy were slight were the worst for the mind, the discharging lesion in such cases being "in the highest and most intellectual of the nervous arrangements" (p. 121).

Hughlings Jackson referred to Falret's writings and gave the following classification of the association between the mental state and epilepsy:

1. The sudden and transient mental disorder after one or a few fits.
2. More lengthy infirmity after a rapid succession of numerous fits.
3. The persistent deterioration, the result of fits repeated for months or years.

He also initially subscribed to the doctrine of masked epilepsy, but expressed doubts. He said: "Epileptic mania, although it usually occurs after a fit . . . sometimes replaces a fit. . . . It has been said that the patient who is subject to attacks in which there is a convulsion of muscles may at another time have an attack in which there is a 'convulsion of ideas,' and corresponding excess of external action. I used to adopt the hypothesis of masked epilepsy. But I do not now think it possible. . . . I think another hypothesis is preferable. I think it probable that there is a transitory epileptic paroxysm in every case of mental automatism" (Taylor, 1958, p. 122).

His explanation for the behaviour was that the epileptic paroxysm had two effects. It resulted in loss of consciousness, with loss of control permitting increased automatic action.

One of Hughlings Jackson's patients, Dr. Z, has recently been the subject of renewed interest (Taylor and Marsh, 1980). Dr. Z was Arthur Thomas Myers, and his case is described in Hughlings Jackson's 1888 paper in *Brain* (Taylor, 1958, p. 385). In this he describes a form of epilepsy in which the "intellectual aura" or "dreamy state" is the striking symptom. His patient and others mentioned in this paper describe what are now recognised as classical symptoms of temporal lobe epilepsy. Dr. Z committed suicide from an overdose of chloral, and at postmortem examination was shown to have a small lesion in the left uncinate gyrus. Although Taylor and Marsh argue that this lesion was most probably an artefact, the case is important for several reasons. Dr. Z helped Hughlings Jackson formulate more clearly this type of seizure and distinguish it from other forms of partial epilepsy. One way Dr. Z helped him was by the habit of recording symptoms in extensive written accounts. In Dr. Z's obituary, published in the *British Medical Journal* of January 27, 1894, we read that he, "with singular patience, minuteness, and fidelity . . . invented a system of indexing. . . . He was much interested in some of the problems which the 'psychical researchers' aspire to solve. . . . His history is tinged by a touch of melancholy. . . . destiny thought fit to inflict upon him that terrible and inscrutable nervous malady which occasionally harassed him in early youth, and of late years advanced with relentless dread, baffling the most devoted medical skill and ultimately involving a fine intellect in ruin and confusion."

It is further known that he never married and had an interest in the mystical. His last paper was 50 pages long and titled "Mind-cure, Faith-cure and Miracles of Lourdes." Is it possible that we have here a description of the kind of person referred to as having epileptic personality changes? Is Dr. Z, with his hypergraphia, obsession, and religiosity, an exemplum of the characteristics of the Geschwind syndrome? (see p. 119).

Another English author to discuss epilepsy and its consequences was Maudsley (1835–1918). He was especially interested in the forensic aspects of mental disease, and the question of individual responsibility. He described epileptic mania, "a most dangerous form of insanity," in which:

in a frenzy of excitement, unconscious of what he is doing, his senses perhaps possessed with frightful hallucinations, he is driven to most destructive acts of violence against both animate and inanimate objects (Maudsley, 1874, p. 228).

He went on to describe the progression of epilepsy:

> There may be no impairment whatever at first, although after the disease has lasted for some time there will be a loss of memory and weakness of mind, deepening into actual dementia in the worst cases. It is one of the saddest experiences of asylum life to witness the pitiful fate of those patients who have not sunk below the consciousness of their condition. Gentle, amiable, and industrious through their long intervals of lucidity, they hope against hope that each recurring paroxysm will be the last; they eagerly try all remedies, in the hope of curing the disease; they see others leave the asylum restored to health, and confidently anticipate that their turn will come; but confidence wanes as the attacks recur, the mind is slowly weakened by the storms of fury through which it passes, and they sink finally into the apathy of dementia (p. 228).

Maudsley also accepted the concept of masked epilepsy and that changes of character and temperament could occur months or even years before distinctly epileptic seizures were manifest. He classified the mental disorders of epilepsy into four categories thus:

1. Prodromata or forerunners
2. Those corresponding in the mental sphere to the slight form of epilepsy known as petit mal
3. More violent symptoms that would correspond to regular epileptic convulsions or grand mal
4. Mental decay following long-continued epilepsy.

In type four, Maudsley specifically mentions the development of an exaggerated sentiment, visual hallucinations, and "like Swedenborg, they are sometimes carried up into heaven while yet in the flesh, and have conferences with the Supreme" (p. 243).

Such religiosity was the subject of a study by Howden (1873). He set out to describe "a feature in the mental condition of epileptics" which he felt was not uncommon. He recognised these "strong devotional feelings" which manifest either as simple piety or religious delusions. Several case histories were provided, emphasising differing shades of religiosity, and some support provided for the concept that "many religious fanatics were epileptics." The latter included Mohammed, Ann Lee (the mother of the Shakers) and Swedenborg.

Passages from the novels of Dostoievski, notably from *The Idiot and The Possessed*, are also reminiscent of some of these characteristics. Dostoievski was known to have epilepsy, and had personally experienced ecstatic moments. These have been described by his friend Trakhov as follows: "Fyodor Mikhailovitch on several occasions spoke to me of periods of exultation which preceded an attack. He said that 'for several brief moments I feel a contentedness which is unthinkable under normal conditions, and unimaginable for those who have not experienced it. At such times I am in perfect harmony with myself and with the entire universe. Perception is so clear and so agreeable that one would give 10 years of this life, and perhaps all of it for a few seconds of such bliss' (Gastaut, 1978).

Dostoievski is also reported as saying: "I had the feeling that the sky had descended to the ground and had swallowed me up. I truly felt the presence of God, and he entered into me."

The saintly Prince Myshkin had similar auras in *The Idiot*.

THE GERMAN CONTRIBUTION

Towards the end of the nineteenth century, the medical hegemony moved away from France to Germany. Neuropsychiatry was no exception, and a number of German writers took an interest in epilepsy. A starting point is the work of Griesinger (1817–1868). He was a professor of psychiatry and neurology in Berlin and clearly formulated the idea that normal mental processes are dependent on brain function, and that the latter was involved in insanity. His dictum was: "Insanity being a disease, and that disease being an affection of the brain, it can therefore only be studied in a proper manner from the medical point of view" (Griesinger, 1857, p. 9).

He recognised epilepsy as a cause of insanity, both acutely and chronically. He also suggested that psychical disturbances could occur before the epilepsy was manifest, and in established cases alternating with epileptic attacks. He noted that "a very great number of epileptics are in a state of chronic mental disease even during the intervals between attacks." He used the term *psychomotor symptoms* and accepted the idea that psychoses could substitute for seizures as shown in the following case history:

CASE I.

A peasant, born at Krumbach in Swabia, age 27, and unmarried, was subject from his eighth year to epileptic attacks. Two years ago, his disease changed its character without any one being able to account for it; and in place of epileptic attacks, the man found himself seized [sic] by an irresistible disposition to commit murder. He feels the approach of the fit several hours, and sometimes a day, before it comes on. Immediately when he has the presentiment, he earnestly asks to be tied up and bound with chains, lest he commit some crime.

He feels himself greatly exhausted, and experiences slight convulsive movements in the limbs. . . . The fit lasts one to two days (Griesinger, 1857, p. 297).

Griesinger's pupil, Horing, produced a dissertation on automatisms, and elaborated on the concept of incompletely developed epilepsy, with minimal change of consciousness and few, if any, convulsions.

The term *epileptic equivalent* seems to have first been used by Hoffmann in 1862. He noted, in a short paper, that "eventually epileptic seizures may be missed completely, but the mental disease can reveal, through its particular symptoms and signs, that it is an equivalent of epilepsy, especially of convulsions and coma."

Samt (1875, 1876), a psychiatrist from Berlin, elaborated the concept of epileptic equivalents in a study of over 40 cases. His classification of epileptic insanity recognised two major forms, namely, psychic equivalents and postepileptic insanity. Psychic equivalents were recognised by their clinical form which included episodes of violence, religious ecstasy, anxious delirium, and stupor.

Kraepelin (1856–1925), professor of psychiatry at Munich and Heidelberg, whose work on classification has so profoundly influenced psychiatry in the twentieth century, also studied epileptic insanity. He recognised the latter as one of the major forms of mental illness, alongside dementia praecox and manic depressive illness. He quotes Samt with approval, recognising the pleomorphic forms of epileptic symptoms. He described cases of epileptic delirium, with religious hallucinations and delusions, and emphasised how alcohol might exacerbate the psychopathology (Kraepelin, 1904). He drew much attention to the acute mood changes of epilepsy which may be associated with more prolonged episodes of hallucinations and delusions. This state, he noted, may bear some resemblance to dementia praecox.

The periodic mood swings seen in patients with epilepsy were further discussed by Aschafferberg (1906). He reported that 70% of his cases had such fluctuations of mood, with no obvious relationship to their seizures. The attacks had a sudden onset and termination without obvious cause, although they could be induced by small amounts of alcohol. Such mood swings were also noted by Gaupp (1903).

It was a short step to the concepts of such authors as Bratz and Leubuscher (1907) who defined *affect epilepsy*, attacks precipitated by psychological factors which consisted of loss of consciousness, dizziness, hallucinations, and rage.

The position at the end of the nineteenth century is best summed up by reference to Savage's (1892) contribution to Tuke's *Dictionary of Psychological Medicine*. He accepted the hereditary principle, and that epilepsy "is a most important factor in the production" of insanity. He noted preictal, ictal, and interictal associations, and noted that before a seizure, "brief attacks of insanity, generally of a maniacal type" may be seen. He accepted the concept of masked epilepsy and speculated on its pathogenesis: "In the two classes of cases [seizures, and impulsive destructive acts without convulsions], similar discharges of nerve force along paths of least resistance take place and may become habitual by recurrence; the difference is slight, whether there be a discharge of motor force, which is altogether purposeless or whether there be a discharge, which, though unconscious, is still along certain definite lines, which may have been by use established" (p. 453).

Postictal automatisms were a well-recognised cause of insanity, and he thought that many cases of so-called masked epilepsy fell into this class. The postepileptic symptoms were often violent, in many cases being epileptic mania, although melancholia was another variant. This was usually associated with ideas of persecution and strong religious tendencies.

Savage was of the opinion that successive attacks led to a gradual weakening of the mind, with dementia being the inevitable outcome.

THE NATURE OF THE LINK; THE TWENTIETH CENTURY

Along with these presentations of the clinical nature of epileptic insanity and its variants, there was much speculation on the nature of the link. To understand this, it is important to note that in the nineteenth century there was considerable discussion on the nature of mental illness and the differing forms of insanity.

For some, such as Griesinger, there was only one major psychosis (Einheitpsychose). The disorder changed its manifestations over time, but what were viewed were only different stages of the same morbid process. Others, for example, Kraepelin, defined several forms, all thought related to differing underlying disease states. Since by the end of the nineteenth century many writers recognised that epilepsy and insanity were somehow interlinked, the nature of this relationship became a matter for debate. Berrios (1979) has reviewed this, providing the following summary of the prevailing views:

1. The link as a chance combination:
   A.) as the result of defective statistics (Herpin)
   B.) as the result of a chance genetic combination (Magnan)

2. The link as real:
   A.) epilepsy producing psychosis
      i) by disrupting reality testing (Ziehen; Gaupp)
      ii) by weakening the brain (Bucholz)
   B.) psychosis producing epilepsy (Clouston)
   C.) both being the result of a common organic factor (Hughlings Jackson)

In the main, these hypotheses have been the ones considered over time, and these issues are further discussed in later chapters of this book. Some further clarification, however, is necessary. Magnan (1835–1912), a pupil of Falret, took up the principles of Morel (1809–1873): that degenerative hereditary strains were pathological variations which would get worse from one generation to the next. Epilepsy would be considered one reflection of such degeneration and, as Hill (1981) has pointed out, these ideas had a long-lasting influence on psychiatry, but also influenced ideas about epilepsy. They were associated with the unitary view of psychosis, led to ideas of a constitutional predisposition to epilepsy based on personality features (see p. 109), and contributed to the continuing stigma attached to epilepsy by both the general public and the medical profession.

Morel's view was taken up by Maudsley (1879) and expressed as follows: "When epilepsy in young children leads to idiocy, as it often does, we must generally look for the deep root of the mischief in the family neurosis. . . . Epilepsy in the parent may engender the insane neurosis in the child, and insanity in the parent the epileptic neurosis in the child" (pp. 45, 65).

Another British physician influenced by these theories was Aldren Turner (1907), physician to the National Hospital, Queen Square, and consultant to the Colony for Epileptics, Chalfont Saint Peter, as it was then called. Turner wrote: "In epilepsy, as in other degenerative neuroses, stigmata of degeneration are present . . . [these] are deviations from the normal, and occur in those who are subjects of a hereditary degenerative predisposition" (p. 17).

For Magnan, the combinations and metamorphic relationship between epilepsy and psychotic episodes were explained by the concept of double inheritance: one parent contributing to epilepsy, the other to the insanity.

The idea that a person could suffer from two psychoses led to discussion of the nature of the relationship between them. Stransky (1906) pointed out that one must separate the simultaneous from the successive; others questioned the pathoplastic effects of the one on the other (Gaupp, 1903; Glaus, 1931). The question of whether or not the psychosis produced epilepsy or vice versa was answered by individual case histories, and as psychiatric terminology changed, the majority of papers concentrated on schizophrenia. The combination of schizophrenia and epilepsy was variously reported as common (Yde, 1941) and rare (Krapf, 1928; Glaus, 1931); the by then well-recorded observation that, in some patients, by the time the psychosis appeared the epilepsy had become quiescent was used as an illustration of the incompatibility of the two psychoses.

If the psychosis brought with it seizures, the latter was viewed as part of the schizophrenic process, while various theories were put forward to explain how the epilepsy could damage the brain to lead to the psychosis, including via raised intracranial pressure, autointoxication, and endocrine disturbances. Others preferred more psychological explanations; for example, that the recurrent psychic disorganisation of the ictus could lead to chronic illness (Ziehen, 1902).

CONCLUSIONS

It has been shown that associations between epilepsy and mental illness have been observed since antiquity. The most important era, historically, is the nineteenth century, most notably with the observations of the mid-century French alienists and German neuropsychiatrists. All of the arguments that still pervade this subject can be seen to have been rehearsed over the ensuing decades, including the possibility that all are based on observational and statistical artefacts due to patients being observed and collected in the asylum setting.

The concept of epileptic equivalents had a profound effect on this debate. There can be no doubt that this idea was accepted by many highly experienced and influential physicians such as Aldren Turner. As a topic, it fell from favour in the early part of the twentieth century, but by then the notion had transmogrified into an acceptance of and an explanation for interictal personality changes and hence psychoses. Further, it accounted for other paroxysmal clinical phenomena that may not even be associated with seizures, or a history of them, that were often of a violent nature.

It seems to be the case that often observations of the coadunation of epilepsy and insanity were made by neuropsychiatrists in an asylum setting, although this was not always so. Kraepelin was not an asylum physician, and Hughlings Jackson was a neurologist. Those who denied the association had, like Reynolds, to remove insane patients from their own statistics.

The debate over the association between epilepsy and schizophrenia moderated in the first half of the twentieth century, especially as the view that it was rare seems to have become established (see Chapter 5). A resurgence of interest occurred in the 1950s, the literature from which time is reviewed in other chapters of this book.

2

Epilepsy and Its Classification

SOME THEORETICAL ISSUES

The process of classification in medicine is not the empirical science it is often thought to be. It was Hughlings Jackson who pointed out that, in general, there are two kinds of classifiers: the gardener and the botanist, and that physicians tend to be gardeners. He accepted that the gardener's arrangement was better than that of the botanist for some purposes. He also noted: "Because it is convenient to consider a whale as a fish for legal purposes, it would never do to consider it so in zoology" (Taylor, 1958, p. 288).

Epilepsy and the psychoses that we are considering are essentially clinical phenomena, and the terms imply nothing specific in regard to aetiology (the underlying cause) and pathogenesis (the mechanism whereby that cause leads to symptomatology).

It is customary in clinical practice to assume that disease has some independent existence of its own, visiting our healthy bodies and altering them in some way. Physicians note these changes, establish the pattern that they assume, ascribe a diagnosis, and prescribe a remedy which will influence the unwanted guest. Earlier theories of this model attributed disease to the intrusion of spirits and evil forces, often seen as punishment for wrongdoing. Epilepsy was viewed in this way and still is by some cultures. The idea that disease is due to intrusion from outside agencies was given a boost by the discovery of microorganisms, and their cure by antibiotics led some to believe that diseases would all have a single cause and, ideally, a single treatment.

However, a number of other concepts of disease must be considered which are of importance for an understanding of the relationship between epilepsy and psychosis. For the Platonists, health was seen as a state of harmony, and loss of this resulted in pain and disease. Since the elements that made up the body were the same as those that constituted the universe, theories of causation were based not on observation, but on the Platonic perception of the universe. Alternative themes are reflected in models of disease that assume the existence of disease as an objective reality, but embrace notions of aetiology that intertwine the nature of the disease with the relationship of man to nature. Diseases have thus been attributed to the increasing or decreasing influence of civilisation and the evils of "modern society." A forerunner of these ideas comes from the writings of Rousseau (1712–1778), whose dislike for the evils of "civilisation" included the consequent induced diseases. Some current ideas stress the evils of industrialisation as both aetiological and pathogenic for psychiatric illness and, in some patients' minds, for epilepsy.

Hippocrates (460–377 BC) introduced the historical dimension to disease and the first medical case histories were from this era. The disease had signs and symptoms, a beginning, a course, and an outcome. This view is often lost sight of, particularly in clinical practice where delineation of current signs and symptoms takes so much precedence over history gathering. Nonetheless, the diagnosis of epilepsy, of psychosis, and of the relationship of the two can often only be discerned by careful anamnesis.

The step to recognising diseases as independent entities came in the seventeenth century with the works of Baglivi (d. 1707) and Sydenham (1624–1689). They felt that diseases in their natural states were subject to the same laws of observation and description as other natural phenomena. The final step was made by Virchow (1821–1902), who combined his cellular pathology with the new knowledge of anatomicoclinical medicine, completing the notion of disease as a local affection. The search for classification systems as well as aetiology became predominant.

Entwined with the development of the concept of disease as an independent local entity has been the important principle of reaction. Sydenham (1740) recognised this when he said: "A disease is nothing else but nature's endeavour to thrust forth with all her might the morphic matter for the health of the patient" (p. 1).

Thus, intrinsic as well as extrinsic factors assume importance in the pathogenesis of symptoms. The reactions of the organism were seen as healing; an extension of this thinking is described by Riese (1953): "A disease is a whole of vital manifestations, elicited by some pathogenic (extrinsic) factor or groups of them, and displayed by organisms whose reactions, though similar in some respects, differ from individual to individual" (p. 39).

This biographic conception of disease stands in obvious contrast to the ontological one in the sense that it admits only diseased individuals and not diseases per se.

Hughlings Jackson, in his paper on the "factors of insanities," cites four. They all pertain to dissolution. The second is "different persons who have undergone dissolution," while the fourth is "the influence . . . of different external circumstances on the persons who have undergone that dissolution" (Taylor, 1958, p. 143). In other words, the final pattern of symptoms is dependent in some disorders as much upon the brain of the person affected and its experience as upon any disease factors per se. This conception of disease has had a marked influence on psychiatry, where ultimately the testimony of individuals, as opposed to clinical observation, assumed an ever-increasing significance, culminating with the psychoanalytic methods. Further, the phrase "reaction types" became accepted, especially in North America, with the contributions of Adolf Meyer's (1866–1950) *Psychobiology*.

SIGNS, SYMPTOMS, SYNDROMES, AND DISEASE

In clinical medicine there are two fundamental kinds of data. Symptoms are the complaints that the patient tells us about or are elicited by clinical history. Signs are observed by the physician, the patient, or a friend or relative of the patient, which indicate the presence of abnormal functioning of one or more bodily systems. A syndrome is a constellation of signs and symptoms which may coalesce to provide what seems to be a recognisable entity with defining characteristics. Syndromes then become classified, and are the clinical representatives of illness. The latter infers some biological change or variation of the organism, and it is the task of medical science to explore this. However, a clear distinction has to be drawn between illness and disease, and between syndromes and diseases. Illness is that which the patient presents to doctors with, which only represents in part the expression of disease in any individual. Syndromes are not synonymous with diseases, since the same underlying aetiology may provoke a variety of syndromes, while the same syndrome may have differing aetiologies and pathogeneses.

As a consequence, classification of disease in medicine generally represents a variety of notions, and neurology is no exception. Epilepsy is a syndrome or group of syndromes identified by a key symptom, namely, recurrent seizures. Schizophrenia and manic-depressive illness are likewise defined by a collection of symptoms which coalesce into recognisable syndromes. Other states, however, are diagnosed by pathology, for example, Alzheimer's disease; still others relate to a patient's behaviour, for example, hysteria. Indeed, with regard to diseases of the brain, no attempt has been made to provide a comprehensive classification system since that of Romberg (1795–1873) in 1853. It follows from this, however, that two separate syndromes; for example, epilepsy and schizophrenia, may well have similar underlying pathological links, and although they appear different on the surface, they may have more in common than their external manifestations initially suggest.

CLASSIFICATION OF EPILEPSY

In order to explore associations between psychiatric illness and epilepsy, it is necessary to view current classifications in some detail. With regard to epilepsy, even defining it is difficult. The often-quoted definition of Hughlings Jackson: "occasional, sudden, rapid and local discharges of grey matter" (Taylor, 1958, p. 100) emphasises the acute paroxysmal nature of the disorder, but fails to distinguish it from other similar disorders; for example, migraine or acute panic attacks. While it is accepted that the cardinal clinical symptom of epilepsy is the seizure, and it is usual to accept that epilepsy requires recurrent as opposed to a single seizure before a diagnosis can be made, it has to be emphasised that epilepsy, like schizophrenia, refers to a heterogenous group of conditions in which clear evidence for organic brain dysfunction becomes evident the more it is looked for. However, even with modern technology, recurrent seizures often occur in the absence of identifiable neuropathology.

EARLIER CLASSIFICATIONS

It was Cullen (1712–1790) who laid a framework for classificiation of disease which has had influence up to the present day. He described four main classes, one being the neuroses. These included "all those preternatural affections of sense and motion which are without pyrexia as part of the primary disease . . . but depend on a more general affection of the nervous system, and of those powers of the system upon which sense and motion more especially depend" (Cullen, 1800).

In this scheme convulsions and epilepsy were classified under the subcategory "Spasmi," along with, for example, hysteria, hydrophobia, colic, and chorea. The epilepsies were themselves subdivided into idiopathic and sympathetic groups, the latter being related to stimulation of the nerves from some part of the body which then in sympathy affects the brain. Pinel (1745–1826), a follower of Cullen and translator of some of his works into French, defined epilepsy as a neurosis of cerebral function; Pinel's pupil, Maisonneuve, distinguished ten different species of epilepsy, five idiopathic and five sympathetic.

In Romberg's classification there were two major groupings, namely, the neurosis of sensibility and the neurosis of motility. Epilepsy belonged to the latter. Gradually, these classifications based on function became replaced by those based on supposed aetiology, and the concept of epileptiform convulsions, in which there was an established disease of the brain present, became clarified. Hughlings Jackson introduced evolutionary concepts into his classifications, referring to lowest level fits as "pontobulbar," middle level fits as "epileptiform," while highest level fits were "epileptic." Of more importance in Hughlings Jackson's writing, however, was his clear delineation of the concept of partial epilepsy. Similar ideas were first elaborated by Prichard (1786–1848) (1822), who wrote of "local convulsion or partial epilepsy," identifying examples of epilepsy without convulsions. Todd (1809–1860) (1856) used the term *epileptiform* for attacks that affected one arm or leg or both on the same side. Hughlings Jackson more fully described the clinical features of such partial episodes, which were ultimately designated "Jacksonian" by the French neurologist Charcot (1825–1893). Hughlings Jackson thus stated in his "Study of convulsions" (Taylor, 1958) that the great majority of convulsions could be arranged into two classes: those in which the spasm affected both sides of the body almost contemporaneously and those in which the fit began by deliberate spasm on one side of the body and in which parts of the body were affected one after another. The former were referred to as "idiopathic epilepsy," although the term "genuine" was also given to this grouping.

Hughlings Jackson also introduced us to another very important group of seizures. These he referred to as patients who had a particular variety of epilepsy with "intellectual aura" (Taylor, 1958, p. 385). Patients reported "dreamy states," with alteration of their mental state (Hughlings Jackson's important case, Dr. Z, has already been referred to in Chapter 1). It was upon such cases that the idea arose that a seizure could occur with minimal or no motor components, and primarily affect the mental state. Since pathological lesions in some of these cases at postmortem examination were described in the "uncinate lobe" of the temporal cortex, they were referred to as "the uncinate group of fits."

In this century, little attempt was made to classify epilepsy any further until the introduction into clinical practice of the electroencephalogram (EEG) in the 1940s, which allowed classification to be based on observed changes in electrical activity in the brain during a seizure. This advance, however, highlighted an important principle: namely, that seizures, the symptom of epilepsy, can be more readily classified than epilepsy itself. A second principle was the clear recognition of the existence of symptomatic epilepsies related to cortical lesions and a broad delineation of seizures into those of generalised onset and those of focal onset. Gibbs et al. (1938) considered that epilepsy could be classified into three main groups, namely, grand mal, petit mal, and psychomotor. The term *temporal lobe epilepsy* was introduced shortly thereafter, but neither the term *psychomotor*, nor *temporal lobe epilepsy* added much to what had originally been described by Hughlings Jackson.

Penfield and Jasper (1954) retained the terms *symptomatic* and *idiopathic*, but from their own work derived an anatomicoclinical classification, suggesting that it was important to recognise whether attacks arise from the cerebral cortex or from the subcortical region, the latter being defined as centrencephalic. These then become subdivided into several types, dependent on their EEG patterns, which included petit mal, grand mal, and "psychomotor automatisms." Focal, or partial, epilepsies became a crucial area of investigation opened up by the EEG, and the clarification of primary and secondary generalised seizures occurred, as did clear recognition that the symptoms evoked in focal epilepsy were dependent upon the site of origin within the brain of the abnormal discharge.

In more recent times there have been attempts to revise classifications of both seizures and epilepsy. The classification of seizures has been more successful, catalysed by the development of video telemetry, during which investigations patients' seizures can be viewed alongside their individual EEG patterns. The apparent success at classifying seizures, however, has not been echoed with the classification of the epilepsies.

RECENT CLASSIFICATIONS

Seizures

The revised International League Against Epilepsy (ILAE) classification of epileptic seizures (1981) is shown in Table 2.1. Partial seizures are those in which the clinical and EEG changes suggest a focal onset, and the classification is based

TABLE 2.1. *Revised ILAE Classification of Epileptic Seizures*

I   Partial (focal, local) seizures
   A   Simple partial seizures (consciousness not impaired)
   B   Complex partial seizures (with impairment of consciousness: may sometimes begin
      with simple symptomatology)
   C   Partial seizures evolving to secondarily generalised seizures (this may be generalised
      tonic-clonic, tonic, or clonic)
II   Generalised seizures (convulsive or nonconvulsive)
III   Unclassified epileptic seizure

(International League Against Epilepsy, 1981)

mainly on whether or not consciousness is impaired in the attack. In a simple partial seizure, consciousness is retained. Various forms are recognised; for example, with focal motor seizures, which when accompanied by a march are referred to as Jacksonian; with somatosensory or special sensory symptoms; with autonomic symptoms; or associated with psychic symptoms such as dysphasia, dysmnesia (for example, déjà vu), cognitive, affective, illusory, or hallucinatory experiences. In general, this last group of symptoms is often accompanied by impairment of consciousness, and is therefore more associated with complex partial seizures. In the latter, impairment of consciousness is often the first clinical sign, although a simple partial seizure may evolve into the complex variety. In patients presenting to psychiatric clinics, complex partial seizures are the most common seizure type, and patients usually (but not inevitably) give a history of progression to generalised motor seizures on occasions.

Generalised seizures are those in which the first clinical changes suggest bilateral abnormalities with widespread disturbances of both hemispheres. Absence seizures (petit mal) are usually associated with regular 3 Hz per second spike and slow wave activity on the EEG, although variants of this with 2–3 Hz activity may be seen. Tonic-clonic seizures are the classical grand mal attacks associated with accompanying EEG abnormalities.

As investigation of the brains of patients with epilepsy becomes more precise, it has become clear that many seizures previously diagnosed as generalised are in fact partial seizures, especially from frontal cortices which have secondarily generalised. This has considerable significance for investigations that have traditionally divided patients into those with partial and generalised attacks, as it is most likely the case that, in many, the generalised seizures were essentially derived from a focus.

It should be noted that in this latest classification, the term *complex* has been altered from an earlier classification. In the 1969 version, the term *complex* was used to refer to alteration of higher cortical function and had some neuroanatomical logic, in the sense of implying altered function of the integrative cortices of the brain, stemming from the work of Penfield. The newer classification is based solely on clinical phenomenology and, therefore, loses a potentially important ingredient with regard to brain–behaviour associations, namely, anatomical localisation.

Epilepsies

Although approximately 1 in 20 people may be susceptible to have a seizure during their lifetime, the prevalence of epilepsy is far less, being around 0.5% for the general population. A provisional classification of the epilepsies has recently been published (International League Against Epilepsy, 1985). This is essentially a classification of syndromes rather than diseases, and an abbreviated version is shown in Table 2.2.

Terms found in earlier versions, such as *primary* and *secondary*, have been omitted, and the main dichotomy separates epilepsies with generalised seizures from those with partial or focal seizures, the latter being referred to as localisation-related partial or focal epilepsies. Of particular relevance here are the localisation-related symptomatic seizures, further designated by the area of localisation affected. Under temporal lobe epilepsies there are subdivisions, with particular emphasis on hippocampal and amygdalar pathology. These epilepsies characteristically present with partial seizures, alteration of consciousness, and often automatisms.

TOWARDS A DEFINITION OF LIMBIC EPILEPSY

It was probably Fulton who first suggested that the term *limbic epilepsy* should be applied to seizures arising from medial temporal structures (Glaser, 1967). He said, "Temporal lobe seizures . . . might more properly be designated as seizures involving the limbic lobe" (Fulton, 1953).

The concept was more fully developed by Glaser (1967), who entitled a paper "Limbic Epilepsy in Childhood," in which 12 children were described who had "psychomotor seizures" with minimal secondary generalisation. In common terminology all would be described as suffering from complex partial seizures, and the majority of them suffered interictal behaviour disorders. These were mainly personality disturbances of varying degrees, but eight had psychotic reactions with schizophrenia-like disturbances, and the development of paranoid, delusional, and hallucinatory symptoms. Glaser pointed out the high susceptibility of limbic system structures to pathological processes, including ischemia, encephalitis, and meta-

---

TABLE 2.2. *ILAE Classification of Epilepsies*

---

1. Localisation-related (focal, local, partial) epilepsies and syndromes
     Idiopathic with age-related onset (e.g., benign epilepsy of childhood)
     Symptomatic (e.g., frontal lobe, temporal lobe)
2. Generalised epilepsies or syndromes
     Idiopathic
     Idiopathic and/or symptomatic (e.g., West's syndrome)
     Symptomatic
3. Epilepsies and syndromes undetermined as to whether they are focal or generalised
4. Special syndromes (e.g., febrile convulsions)

(International League Against Epilepsy, 1985)

bolic disturbances, and suggested that the term *psychomotor* or *temporal lobe* should give way to the designation "limbic" when this form of epilepsy was described.

This idea represents the full development of a concept elaborated by Hughlings Jackson many years previously. Following his papers, little seems to have been written about this form of epilepsy until Gibbs and colleagues (1937) introduced us to "psychomotor epilepsy," which was associated with observed abnormalities from the temporal lobe on the EEG. Jasper and colleagues (1951) introduced the term *temporal lobe seizures* to denote such focal seizures. This embraced a wide variety of focal seizure patterns, from the uncinate seizure of Jackson to the psychomotor seizure of Gibbs and colleagues. Temporal lobe epilepsy became synonymous with psychomotor epilepsy, which led to a considerable confusion, not the least because a psychomotor seizure could arise from areas outside the temporal lobes, and patients with temporal lobe epilepsy presented with seizure types other than that classified as psychomotor. Further, the confusion between the classification of epilepsy and the classification of seizures was not well appreciated at that time.

The developing neuroanatomical and neurochemical techniques of the 1940s and 1950s and animal ablation and stimulation experiments focused more sharply on differences of both structure and function between the medial temporal structures and their associated limbic circuits, and those of the neocortical temporal lobe with its extensive cortico-cortical connections. The idea that temporal lobe seizures could thus properly be subdivided into at least two categories, one being identified by limbic system origin, was an obvious step. Girgis (1981) recommended adoption of the term *limbic epilepsy* as a substitute for both psychomotor and temporal lobe epilepsy, an idea formulated in a proposed earlier version of the ILAE classification of terminology of the epilepsies. Thus, the initial proposed classification, as opposed to the version shown in Table 2.2, included the term *limbic epilepsy* as one of the subdivisions.

The further breakdown is shown in Table 2.3, the overall subdivisions being

TABLE 2.3. *Classification of the Epilepsies*

Localization-related symptomatic epilepsies	
Frontal	Supplementary motor
	Cingulate
	Polar (anterior)
	Orbitofrontal
	Dorsolateral
	Motor cortex
Temporal	Hippocampal (mesiobasal limbic)
	Amygdalar
	Lateral posterior
	Opercular (insular)
Parietal	
Occipital	

(International League Against Epilepsy, 1985)

frontal lobe epilepsies, temporal lobe epilepsies, parietal epilepsies, and occipital lobe epilepsy. Within the temporal lobe group there are hippocampal, amygdalar, lateral posterior and opercular subgroups. The hippocampal group is also labelled "mediobasal limbic" or "primary rhinencephalic psychomotor" epilepsy. Within this classification it can clearly be contrasted with the lateral posterior temporal group, and distinctions are given as shown in Table 2.4.

The hippocampal epilepsies are said to comprise about 70 to 80% of temporal lobe epilepsies, and are commonly combined together with amygdalar epilepsies. The seizures are complex focal seizures associated with an aura, hallucinations or illusions, a motionless stare (arrest), and oral or alimentary automatisms. The amygdalar seizures are characterised by a rising epigastric sensation, autonomic signs, and often an aura of fear or panic with olfactory or gustatory hallucinations. Oral or alimentary automatisms also occur with this group. In contrast, lateral temporal epilepsy is represented by seizures characterised by auras of auditory or visual perceptual hallucinations, or a language disorder. If they arise in the dominant hemisphere, there may be postictal dysphasia, disturbed orientation, or prolonged auditory hallucinations. It will be noted later (Chapter 6) how the experiential aspects of such seizures are dependent on limbic system stimulation, thus suggesting the subdivisions given in the ILAE classification must not be taken too rigidly. Nonetheless, the principle is given that there are differences between medial (limbic) seizures arising from the hippocampus or amygdala, and the lateral seizures with a cortical onset. There is reason to believe that limbic epilepsy is identifiable and should be separated from other localisation-related seizure disorders. The extensive neuroanatomical and neurochemical distinctions between the medial and lateral temporal areas will be discussed in Chapter 4. It is emphasised how the hippocampus and amygdala integrate information derived from sensory input from the external world, reaching them via a cascading system of projections from primary sensory cortex to the entorhinal cortex and hence to the medial temporal structures,

TABLE 2.4. *Lateral and Mediobasal Limbic Epilepsies*

Lateral	Mediobasal
Phenomenology:	
auditory hallucinations	hallucinations
visual illusions or hallucinations	illusions
aphasia	indescribable feelings
	motionless stare
	oral and alimentary automatisms
	learning and memory problems
EEG:	
midposterior temporal spikes	anterior temporal sharp waves
Common Pathologies:	
trauma	MTS infections
gliomas	
A-V malformations	

(International League Against Epilepsy, 1985)

with knowledge of the internal state of the organism provided by connections to and from the limbic forebrain, the hypothalamus, and descending and ascending brain-stem pathways. The known role of limbic structures in the modulation of emotion and as the site of origin of seizures in many patients provides an obvious anatomical and neurophysiological substrate for an understanding of psychopathology found associated with temporal lobe epilepsy, which is the major theme of this book.

3

Classification of Psychiatric Illness

The two main diagnostic systems in use at the present time are: the International Classification of Diseases (ICD), which derives from the World Health Organization, and the American Psychiatric Association's Diagnostic and Statistical Manual of Mental Disorders (Third Edition, Revised) (DSM-III-R). It is important to emphasise that, although diagnostic fashion changes frequently, some of the categories that we use today were recognised by many earlier generations and have a degree of constancy in time.

Plato recognised three kinds of madness; namely, melancholia, mania, and dementia; madness being equated to loss of reason (Zilboorg, 1941). His personality types were based on the humoural theories that were recognised by the Greeks. Aretaeus seems to have acknowledged that mania and melancholia were somehow related, recognised that senile mental disorders were distinct, and described links between certain temperaments and mental illness.

The first comprehensive classification was that of Cullen (1800). He included under the neuroses a subgroup called "vesaniae", which were disorders of intellectual function without pyrexia or coma. It included: amentia, or imbecility of judgement, which may be present from birth or come on in old age; melancholia; mania; and oneirodynia—disturbed imagination during sleep. Pinel (1806) introduced a system of classification including melancholia, mania, dementia, and idiotism. In Germany, Griesinger (1857) recognised states of mental depression, states of mental exultation, and states of mental weakness.

Gradually, some newer categories of illness became recognised. J-P Falret (1794–1870), father of Jules, described alternating moods of mania and melancholia (*folie circulaire*); hebephrenia was described by Hecker (1843–1909) in 1871; and Kahlbaum (1823–1899) introduced catatonia in 1874. Morel used the term *démence précoce* for a dementing-like condition that affected young people, which was to reappear as Kraepelin's "dementia praecox."

The word *psychosis* seems to have been first used in 1844 by von Feuchtersleben with a rather general meaning (Pichot, 1983), and confusion has surrounded its use ever since.

Kraepelin's textbook of psychiatry went through nine editions, and his views moulded with time and experience. Prognosis was an essential feature of his system, and this was related to diagnosis. Dementia praecox and manic-depressive psychosis were his two main groupings, involutional melancholia and paranoia being considered as separate entities. Three forms of dementia praecox were described; namely, the hebephrenic, the catatonic, and the paranoid. These fundamental categories of psychopathology form the framework of the system in use today. These ideas of Kraepelin were opposed to the unitary psychosis model, and were influential in reaffirming the disease concept in psychiatry.

One more distinction should briefly be discussed: that of the endogenous and the exogenous psychoses. The distinction is attributed initially to Mobius (1853–1907) (Lewis, 1971), who introduced a classification based on causes. He distinguished between main and subsidiary causes: if the chief factor was seen to be within the individual it was referred to as endogenous; if it was something which impinged on the individual from without, it was exogenous. Bonhoeffer (1868–1948) developed in 1909 the concept of exogenous reaction types which reflected various ways that the brain responded to injury. This essentially referred to organic insults arising outside the neurones and damaging the brain. He specifically mentioned epilepsy in association with these ideas. The suggestion was that these reaction types were recognisable patterns of symptoms, and he noted: "The forms which these exogenous psychotic reactions take are, first, delirium . . . next come the epileptiform reactions, which may present as states of anxious or frenzied motor excitement, or alternatively as quiet, affectless twilight states" (1909, p. 499).

While the term *exogenous* is rarely used today, and most of the disorders that it reflected would be subsumed under the organic brain syndromes, the concept clearly has relevance for understanding relationships between epilepsy and psychosis. In contrast, the term *endogenous* is widely used, although as Lewis (1971) pointed out, it is often merely a cloak for ignorance. Its introduction was strongly linked to the degeneration theory, and Lewis felt its use "should be openly linked to presumptive evidence of a powerful hereditary factor in causation" (p. 196).

KARL JASPERS

Although Jaspers's *Allgemeine Psychopathologie* was first written in 1913 and went through nine editions, the English translation did not become available until 1963. His approach was strongly empirical in spite of being rooted in the philosophical school of phenomenology.

Influenced by Kant and Husserl, Jaspers developed a methodology for examining the mental state of another person, which, in its purest form, attempts to delineate psychic events as sharply as possible. Phenomenology thus "gives a concrete description of the psychic states which patients actually experience and presents them for observation" (Jaspers, 1963, p. 55). Further, he sharply delineated between form and content in psychopathology, asserting that "from the phenomenological point of view it is only the form that interests us" (p. 58). Central to his theme is the distinction between psychogenic development and organic process; and the dichotomy between understanding (*Verstehen*) and explanation (*Erklären*), what is "meaningful" and what is "causal."

The distinction between what was meaningful and what was causal reflected the "unbridgeable gulf between genuine connections of external causality and psychic connections which can only be called causal by analogy" (p. 301). This distinction is crucial to our understanding of the development of psychopathology, and has bearing on the epileptic psychoses, as will be discussed later. Essentially, Jaspers was interested in connections between events in the phenomenological world, some of which were apparent as one thing emerges from another. This psychic connection is meaningful, and he gave examples of the anger of someone who is attacked and of actions and decisions that evolve from a motive. However, in psychopathology, such understanding or perception of meaningful connections reaches its limits, and phenomena which we cannot understand at all emerge. Here Jaspers relies on causal explanations, the study of objective causal connections. In other words, such phenomena as we observe in the psychoses or in aphasia require the methods of natural science for their interpretation, and their connections can be established empirically. The laws of their relatedness are those of biology, not psychology.

The approach of Jaspers differed from that of Kraepelin in emphasising a descriptive psychopathology rather than focussing on actual diseases. This was continued by Kurt Schneider, who further outlined criteria to distinguish development from process. The construction of such rating scales as the Present State Examination (PSE) of Wing and colleagues (1974) derives from this approach.

CURRENT CLASSIFICATIONS

The classification schemes in use in psychiatry at the present time are based entirely on symptoms. Various operational definitions have been introduced and are widely employed, the basis of which is the completion of a checklist of symptoms, signs, and historical facts which must be satisfied before a diagnosis is made. The two most popular are the Feighner criteria (Feighner et al., 1972) and the DSM-III (American Psychiatric Association (APA), 1980), recently modified to DSM-III-R (APA, 1987). These may be contrasted with the more descriptive classifications given in the ninth edition of ICD, which (ICD-9) came into use in 1979.

In this text, emphasis is given to the DSM-III-R, since, especially in research, it is assuming increasing importance. Although it adopts a multiaxial classification, this is not overemphasised. However, this is in keeping with the distinction drawn by Jaspers between personality disorder and psychiatric illness, development and process. A comprehensive classification is not given, attention being directed at disorders that are of specific relevance for the psychoses of epilepsy.

PERSONALITY DISORDERS

"We see the personality in the particular way an individual expresses himself, in the way he moves, how he experiences and reacts to situations, how he loves, grows jealous, how he conducts his life in general, what needs he has, what are his longings and aims, what are his ideals and how he shapes them, what values guide him and what he does, what he creates and how he acts" (Jaspers, 1963, p. 428).

Thus, it is by the personality traits that we know someone; traits are enduring and give an air of predictability to a person. There are two ways of defining an abnormal personality, either by a statistical method or one based on ideal types. Jaspers preferred the former, also adopted by Kurt Schneider (1959) who defined abnormal personalities as those who "suffer from their abnormality or through whose abnormality society suffers" (p. 4).

A summary of DSM-III-R personality disorder categories is given in Table 3.1.

Antisocial Personality

The term *psychopathic personality* was used by Schneider to embrace several differing abnormal personality patterns, but is generally now used to infer antisocial personality traits. In the ICD-9 it is referred to as manifesting mainly as sociopathy, and *sociopathic personality* is an alternative term. In Feighner's criteria it is one of the few personality disorders described, suggesting its relatively clear delineation. It is characterised by "disregard for social obligations, lack of feeling for others, and impetuous violence or callous unconcern" (ICD-9). It usually becomes apparent in early life, often with conduct disorder at school, and there is a poor work record and marital history. Drug abuse, alcoholism, pathological lying, and prison convictions may be recorded; and sociopaths tend to display more than accepted sexual deviation, somatization, and outbursts of physical violence. A characteristic feature is the

TABLE 3.1. *Personality Disorders from DSM-III-R*[a]

Cluster A		Cluster B		Cluster C	
301.00	Paranoid (337)	301.70	Antisocial (342)	301.82	Avoidant (351)
301.20	Schizoid (339)	301.83	Borderline (346)	301.60	Dependent (353)
301.22	Schizotypal (340)	301.50	Histrionic (348)	301.40	Obsessive compulsive (354)
		301.81	Narcissistic (349)	301.84	Passive aggressive (356)
				301.90	Personality disorder NOS

(American Psychiatric Association, 1987)
[a]Coded on Axis II

tendency to remit over the years, either in early or midadulthood. The criteria are given in Table 3.2.

Obsessive-Compulsive Personality

This is characterised by a lifelong tendency to meticulousness and punctuality. Patients have difficulty in expressing their emotions and tend to check and recheck on their actions. It is better referred to as the anancastic type, which saves confusion with obsessive-compulsive disorder.

Histrionic Personality

The hysterical personality has links to the sociopathic personality, and in many ways is contrasted with the anancastic. Jaspers defined the type thus: "Hysterical personalities crave to appear, both to themselves and others, as more than they are and to experience more than they are ever capable of" (1963, p. 443).

The characteristic traits are excessive dependence; shallow, labile affects; impulsiveness; verbal exaggeration and excessive gestural display; seductiveness in the presence of relative frigidity, and self-dramatisation. There is a tendency to take overdoses of medication or make other attempts to bring self-harm, and there is some association to somatisation.

This type is clearly distinguished from the anancastic personality. In particular, the impulsiveness and tendency to approximate and exaggerate of the hysterical personality stands in contrast to the calculations and deliberations of the anancastic personality. In contrast to sociopaths, who tend to be male, hysterical personalities are more common in females. There are clear overlaps with sociopathic personalities. DSM-III-R prefers the term *histrionic personality disorder* to prevent confusion with hysteria.

Paranoid Personality

This type is distinguished by continued suspiciousness, mistrust, and excessive sensitivity. Jealousy, transient ideas of reference, litigiousness, and a tendency to avoid intimacy are all features, and individuals often take up minor concerns or causes with tenacious vigour, often collecting vast amounts of documentary evidence to support them. The DSM-III-R criteria for this are given in Table 3.3.

Schizoid Personality

The features are of people who have little affective or social contact, with a tendency to detachment and eccentricity. DSM-III-R also has the category "Schizotypal personality disorder." This includes people with "a pervasive pattern of pecu-

TABLE 3.2. *Diagnostic Criteria for Antisocial Personality Disorder from DSM-III-R*

A. Current age at least 18.
B. Evidence of Conduct Disorder with onset before age 15, as indicated by a history of *three* or more of the following:
   (1) was often truant
   (2) ran away from home overnight at least twice while living in parental or parental surrogate home (or once without returning)
   (3) often initiated physical fights
   (4) used a weapon in more than one fight
   (5) forced someone into sexual activity with him or her
   (6) was physically cruel to animals
   (7) was physically cruel to other people
   (8) deliberately destroyed others' property (other than by fire-setting)
   (9) deliberately engaged in fire-setting
  (10) often lied (other than to avoid physical or sexual abuse)
  (11) has stolen without confrontation of a victim on more than one occasion (including forgery)
  (12) has stolen with confrontation of a victim (e.g., mugging, purse-snatching, extortion, armed robbery)
C. A pattern of irresponsible and antisocial behavior since the age of 15, as indicated by at least *four* of the following:
   (1) is unable to sustain consistent work behavior, as indicated by any of the following (including similar behavior in academic settings if the person is a student):
     (a) significant unemployment for six months or more within five years when expected to work and work was available
     (b) repeated absences from work unexplained by illness in self or family
     (c) abandonment of several jobs without realistic plans for others
   (2) fails to conform to social norms with respect to lawful behavior, as indicated by repeatedly performing antisocial acts that are grounds for arrest (whether arrested or not), e.g., destroying property, harassing others, stealing, pursuing an illegal occupation
   (3) is irritable and aggressive, as indicated by repeated physical fights or assaults (not required by one's job or to defend someone or oneself), including spouse- or child-beating
   (4) repeatedly fails to honor financial obligations, as indicated by defaulting on debts or failing to provide child support or support for other dependents on a regular basis
   (5) fails to plan ahead, or is impulsive, as indicated by one or both of the following:
     (a) traveling from place to place without a prearranged job or clear goal for the period of travel or clear idea about when the travel will terminate
     (b) lack of a fixed address for a month or more
   (6) has no regard for the truth, as indicated by repeated lying, use of aliases, or "conning" others for personal profit or pleasure
   (7) is reckless regarding his or her own or others' personal safety, as indicated by driving while intoxicated, or recurrent speeding
   (8) if a parent or guardian, lacks ability to function as a responsible parent, as indicated by one or more of the following:
     (a) malnutrition of child
     (b) child's illness resulting from lack of minimal hygiene
     (c) failure to obtain medical care for a seriously ill child
     (d) child's dependence on neighbors or nonresident relatives for food or shelter
     (e) failure to arrange for a caretaker for young child when parent is away from home
     (f) repeated squandering, on personal items, of money required for household necessities
   (9) has never sustained a totally monogamous relationship for more than one year
  (10) lacks remorse (feels justified in having hurt, mistreated, or stolen from another)
D. Occurrence of antisocial behavior not exclusively during the course of Schizophrenia or Manic Episodes.

(American Psychiatric Association, 1987)

TABLE 3.3. *Diagnostic Criteria for Paranoid Personality Disorder from DSM-III-R*

A. A pervasive and unwarranted tendency, beginning by early adulthood and present in a variety of contexts, to interpret the actions of people as deliberately demeaning or threatening, as indicated by at least *four* of the following:
    (1) expects, without sufficient basis, to be exploited or harmed by others
    (2) questions, without justification, the loyalty or trustworthiness of friends or associates
    (3) reads hidden demeaning or threatening meanings into benign remarks or events, e.g., suspects that a neighbor put out trash early to annoy him
    (4) bears grudges or is unforgiving of insults or slights
    (5) is reluctant to confide in others because of unwarranted fear that the information will be used against him or her
    (6) is easily slighted and quick to react with anger or to counterattack
    (7) questions, without justification, fidelity of spouse or sexual partner
B. Occurrence not exclusively during the course of Schizophrenia or a Delusional Disorder.

(American Psychiatric Association, 1987)

liarities of ideation, appearance, and behavior and deficits in interpersonal relatedness, beginning by early adulthood and present in a variety of contexts, that are not severe enough to meet the criteria for schizophrenia" (p. 340).

MOOD DISORDERS

One of the advantages of the DSM-III classification of mood disorders was the loss of the distinction between endogenous and reactive depression. DSM-III-R has as the essential feature of this group of conditions "a disturbance of mood, accompanied by a full or partial manic or depressive syndrome, that is not due to any other physical or mental disorder" (p. 213). The latter caveat has importance in relationship to this classification of psychopathology and epilepsy, a theme taken up further below.

Subclassification is into bipolar disorders and depressive disorders, the essential feature of the former being the presence of one or more manic or hypomanic episodes. The depressive disorders subdivide into major depression and dysthymia. The latter is a chronic disturbance of mood which fails to meet the criteria for a major depression. A major depressive episode further subdivides into melancholic or chronic.

The main clinical associations in epilepsy are the major depressive episode and dysthymia, although the psychotic conditions are the manias, bipolar disorders, and major depressive episodes with psychotic features.

Clinical Features

The essence of the affective disorders is the change of mood. In depressive states the patient loses vitality, ceases to enjoy life, and usually admits to a loss of emotional well-being. This fundamental change is associated with an alteration of the whole person, reflected in mood, thought, and posture. Concentration difficulties with complaints of poor memory, increased apathy with diminution of movement, and changes of appetite, food intake, and sleep patterns are found. Feelings of anxiety and tension are invariably present, and sometimes, in contrast to a psychomotor retardation, an agitation with indecision and excessive motor activity occurs. In its extreme form, intense aimless pacing is seen. Loss of energy, fatigability, and tiredness are reported, and many symptoms improve as the day passes.

Some patients do not report or underreport the mood changes, and somatic symptoms are the main complaint. These, referable to any system in the body, easily become the focus of attention for patient and physician, and may lead both off into excursions involving a multitude of investigations which are usually negative.

Suicidal thoughts and preoccupations are frequent, as are thoughts of worthlessness and guilt. Crying is not always reported, although should always be asked about, especially in males. Irritability and increased hostility, especially towards loved ones, increases home tensions, as may loss of libido.

In psychotic states there is loss of insight, and delusions and hallucinations may occur. These invariably have a morbid quality and are understood to derive from the changed mood. The delusions may be about death or dying, impoverishment or failure, guilt or damnation. The hallucinations may be auditory, with voices telling of punishment or demanding suicide; or complex visual phenomena, for example, coffins and the dead appearing. Paranoid symptoms are a common accompaniment of severe depressive states, and not uncommonly hide the underlying mood change.

Mania, in contrast, is associated with an increased sense of well-being and euphoria. Again the process is pervasive. There is pressure of speech and flight of ideas, and increased motor activity. Concentration is poor, patients are easily distractible and are often irritable. Sleep and appetite are disturbed, some patients sleeping only very briefly and rising early to pursue their manic activities. In more extreme forms the patient may be very restless, have markedly disordered speech with rhyming, punning, and word play, and mood changing from euphoric to dysphoric.

In the psychosis of manic phases, the delusions are of grandeur, the patient about to spend a fortune he does not possess. Hallucinations are rare but are nearly always mood congruent.

The diagnostic criteria for major depressive episodes and for manic episodes are given in Tables 3.4 and 3.5.

SCHIZOPHRENIC DISORDERS

The use of the plural here emphasises that schizophrenia should properly be viewed as a collection of disorders with differing pathogeneses. This view is not that developed by Kraepelin, who, while acknowledging the differing clinical pictures that may arise, noted the same basic disturbances suggestive of a common

TABLE 3.4. *Diagnostic Criteria for Major Depressive Episode from DSM-III-R*[a]

A. At least five of the following symptoms have been present during the same two-week period and represent a change from previous functioning; at least one of the symptoms is either (1) depressed mood, or (2) loss of interest or pleasure. (Do not include symptoms that are clearly due to a physical condition, mood-incongruent delusions or hallucinations, incoherence, or marked loosening of associations.)
   (1) depressed mood (or can be irritable mood in children and adolescents) most of the day, nearly every day, as indicated either by subjective account or observation by others
   (2) markedly diminished interest or pleasure in all, or almost all, activities most of the day, nearly every day (as indicated either by subjective account or observation by others of apathy most of the time)
   (3) significant weight loss or weight gain when not dieting (e.g., more than 5% of body weight in a month), or decrease or increase in appetite nearly every day (in children, consider failure to make expected weight gains)
   (4) insomnia or hypersomnia nearly every day
   (5) psychomotor agitation or retardation nearly every day (observable by others, not merely subjective feelings of restlessness or being slowed down)
   (6) fatigue or loss of energy nearly every day
   (7) feelings of worthlessness or excessive or inappropriate guilt (which may be delusional) nearly every day (not merely self-reproach or guilt about being sick)
   (8) diminished ability to think or concentrate, or indecisiveness, nearly every day (either by subjective account or as observed by others)
   (9) recurrent thoughts of death (not just fear of dying), recurrent suicidal ideation without a specific plan, or a suicide attempt or a specific plan for committing suicide
B. (1) It cannot be established that an organic factor initiated and maintained the disturbance
   (2) The disturbance is not a normal reaction to the death of a loved one (Uncomplicated Bereavement)[b]
C. At no time during the disturbance have there been delusions or hallucinations for as long as two weeks in the absence of prominent mood symptoms (i.e., before the mood symptoms developed or after they have remitted).
D. Not superimposed on Schizophrenia, Schizophreniform Disorder, Delusional Disorder, or Psychotic Disorder NOS.

(American Psychiatric Association, 1987)
[a]A "Major Depressive Syndrome" is defined as criterion A.
[b]Morbid preoccupation with worthlessness, suicidal ideation, marked functional impairment or psychomotor retardation, or prolonged duration suggest bereavement complicated by Major Depression.

underlying process. Bleuler (1911), who introduced the term *schizophrenia* "to show that the split of the several psychic functions is one of its most important characteristics" (p. 5), extended the range of the psychopathology, and introduced Freudian psychodynamics into his ideas. He suggested that many of the typical symptoms were determined by "psychic" causes, and distinguished various types, including primary, secondary, and basic. The symptoms delineated by Kraepelin were for Bleuler mainly secondary, derived by a reaction of the sick mind to the illness, primary ones being directly caused by the disease process. Basic symptoms, present at all times, were alteration of affect and volition, ambivalence, and autism. His primary symptoms included bodily symptoms such as muscular excitability and cerebral ones such as slowing of mental processes.

TABLE 3.5. *Diagnostic Criteria for Manic Episode from DSM-III-R*[a]

A. A distinct period of abnormally and persistently elevated, expansive, or irritable mood.

B. During the period of mood disturbance, at least three of the following symptoms have persisted (four if the mood is only irritable) and have been present to a significant degree:
   (1) inflated self-esteem or grandiosity
   (2) decreased need for sleep, e.g., feels rested after only three hours of sleep
   (3) more talkative than usual or pressure to keep talking
   (4) flight of ideas or subjective experience that thoughts are racing
   (5) distractibility, i.e., attention too easily drawn to unimportant or irrelevant external stimuli
   (6) increase in goal-directed activity (either socially, at work or school, or sexually) or psychomotor agitation
   (7) excessive involvement in pleasurable activities which have a high potential for painful consequences, e.g., the person engages in unrestrained buying sprees, sexual indiscretions, or foolish business investments

C. Mood disturbance sufficiently severe to cause marked impairment in occupational functioning or in usual social activities or relationships with others, or to necessitate hospitalization to prevent harm to self or others.

D. At no time during the disturbance have there been delusions or hallucinations for as long as two weeks in the absence of prominent mood symptoms (i.e., before the mood symptoms developed or after they have remitted).

E. Not superimposed on Schizophrenia, Schizophreniform Disorder, Delusional Disorder, or Psychotic Disorder NOS.

F. It cannot be established that an organic factor initiated and maintained the disturbance.[b]

(American Psychiatric Association, 1987)
[a]A "Manic Syndrome" is defined as including criteria A, B, and C. A "Hypomanic Syndrome" is defined as including criteria A and B, but not C, i.e., no marked impairment.
[b]Somatic antidepressant treatment (e.g., drugs, ECT) that apparently precipitates a mood disturbance should not be considered an etiologic organic factor.

An important step was taken by Kurt Schneider. Influenced by both Kraepelin and Jaspers, he was especially concerned with symptoms, and was dissatisfied with the way that Bleuler had introduced such concepts as primary and basic. Schneider introduced the terms *first* and *second rank*, quite different from the divisions of other previous writers. The first rank symptoms, shown in Table 3.6, were introduced for pragmatic diagnostic use, and "if this symptom is present in a non-organic psychosis, then we call that psychosis schizophrenia. . . . the presence of first rank symptoms always signifies schizophrenia" (Schneider, 1957, p. 44). It should be made clear that he accepted that a diagnosis of schizophrenia could be made in the absence of such symptoms; it was their presence that was important. The caveat regarding the presence of an organic disorder is discussed below.

Schneider had no presumption of a common structure for these phenomena, although he discussed them in terms of the lowering of a "barrier" between the self and the surrounding world. Other symptoms were termed "second rank", and were considered much less important for diagnosis.

The first rank symptoms assumed importance for the diagnosis of schizophrenia, especially in the United Kingdom, and were employed widely in research; for example, the PSE being biased to detect them for that diagnostic category. Their

TABLE 3.6. *The First-Rank Symptoms of Schneider*

The hearing of one's thoughts spoken aloud in one's head
The hearing of voices commenting on what one is doing at the time
Voices arguing in the third person
Experiences of bodily influence
Thought withdrawal and other forms of thought interference
Thought diffusion
Delusional perception[a]
Everything in the spheres of feeling, drive and volition which the patient experiences as imposed on him or influenced by others

(Schneider, 1957, p. 43)
[a]An abnormal significance attached to a real perception without any cause that is understandable in rational or emotional terms.

theme is taken up in a later chapter (see p. 130), but their influence on the DSM-III (see below) is clear.

The large multicentre International Pilot Study of Schizophrenia was a transcultural investigation of 1,202 patients in nine countries, including Colombia, Czechoslovakia, Denmark, India, Nigeria, and China in addition to the USSR, the United States, and the United Kingdom (WHO, 1963). The main rating instrument was the PSE, which was acceptable to the patients and clinicians involved, and was shown to possess good reliability. The conclusion was that when psychiatrists diagnose schizophrenia, they have the same condition in mind. Lack of insight, delusional mood, ideas of reference, flatness of affect, auditory hallucinations, and passivity experiences were commonly reported symptoms, and although first rank symptoms were present in only one third, when recorded they almost inevitably led to a diagnosis of schizophrenia.

The first rank symptoms of Schneider have come in for a considerable amount of criticism. The suggestion that their presence is pathognomonic for schizophrenia was advocated mainly by psychiatrists of the Anglo-Saxon school, much less importance being given to them by other European or American schools. In the study of Mellor (1970), 72% of schizophrenic patients in a British sample displayed one or more, and the most common were thought broadcasting (21%), thought insertion (20%), voices arguing (13%), and voices commenting (12%). It has been argued that their detection and boundaries are less clear than they first appear (Koehler, 1979). Further, they do not relate to either heritability (McGuffin et al., 1984) or prognosis (Silverstein and Harrow, 1978).

The ICD-9 refers to the schizophrenic psychoses as a group in which there is a disturbance of the personality, distortion of thinking, delusions, a sense of outside influence, disturbed perception, an abnormal affect out of keeping with reality, and autism. Thought, perception, mood, conduct, and personality are all affected by the same illness, but the diagnosis was not restricted to one with a deteriorating course. The main types recognised were simple, hebephrenic, catatonic, and paranoid, but latent, residual, and schizoaffective types were also included.

The DSM-III-R includes the following as essential features: the presence of cer-

TABLE 3.7. *Psychological Processes Involved in Schizophrenia*

Thought   form*
           content*
Perception*
Affect*
Sense of self*
Volition
Interpersonal functioning*
Psychomotor behaviour*

(American Psychiatric Association, 1987)
*Also involved in seizure disorders.

tain psychotic manifestations during the active phase of the illness and functioning below the highest level previously achieved, characteristic symptoms involving multiple psychological processes, and duration for at least six months. Further, the diagnosis is not made if there is any organic factor involved in the initiation or the maintenance of the disorder.

The characteristic areas of psychological processes involved are shown in Table 3.7, and the full diagnostic criteria are shown in Table 3.8.

Several subtypes are recognised. The disorganised type is characterised by absence of well-systematised delusions, incoherence, and an inappropriate blunted affect associated with mannerisms, social withdrawal, and odd behaviour. This is equated with the hebephrenia of ICD-9. In the catatonic type there is marked motor disturbance, sometimes fluctuating between the extremes of excitement and stupor. The paranoid type denotes prominent persecutory or grandiose delusions or hallucinations, with anger and sometimes violence; the undifferentiated type is for those not classified in these groups; and the residual type is for patients who have a history of at least one past episode, but have minimal psychotic symptoms in the presence of continued evidence of the illness.

The emphasis on recent symptoms detracts from the essential nature of the condition, namely, its tendency to pursue a chronic course, hence the term *dementia praecox*. The history, typically, is of a patient who may or may not have demonstrated early developmental, language, and behavioural problems; who manifests bizarre behaviour in late teens or early adulthood with a deterioration of functioning academically and socially. Although initially a bewildering variety of psychopathological states may be noted, including anxiety, mania, and depression, eventually the longitudinal course of the illness becomes apparent and the psychotic symptoms become manifest.

PARANOID (DELUSIONAL) DISORDERS

The term *paranoid* has been used in psychiatry for many years, but its meaning has shifted from a general expression for madness to a more precise technical ex-

TABLE 3.8. *Diagnostic Criteria for Schizophrenia from DSM-III-R*

A. Presence of characteristic psychotic symptoms in the active phase: either (1), (2), or (3) for at least one week (unless the symptoms are successfully treated):
  (1) two of the following:
    (a) delusions
    (b) prominent hallucinations (throughout the day for several days or several times a week for several weeks, each hallucinatory experience not being limited to a few brief moments)
    (c) incoherence or marked loosening of associations
    (d) catatonic behavior
    (e) flat or grossly inappropriate affect
  (2) bizarre delusions (i.e., involving a phenomenon that the person's culture would regard as totally implausible, e.g., thought broadcasting, being controlled by a dead person)
  (3) prominent hallucinations [as defined in (1)(b) above] of a voice with content having no apparent relation to depression or elation, or a voice keeping up a running commentary on the person's behavior or thoughts, or two or more voices conversing with each other
B. During the course of the disturbance, functioning in such areas as work, social relations, and self-care is markedly below the highest level achieved before onset of the disturbance (or, when the onset is in childhood or adolescence, failure to achieve expected level of social development).
C. Schizoaffective Disorder and Mood Disorder with Psychotic Features have been ruled out, i.e., if a Major Depressive or Manic Syndrome has ever been present during an active phase of the disturbance, the total duration of all episodes of a mood syndrome has been brief relative to the total duration of the active and residual phases of the disturbance.
D. Continuous signs of the disturbance for at least six months. The six-month period must include an active phase (of at least one week, or less if symptoms have been successfully treated) during which there were psychotic symptoms characteristic of Schizophrenia (symptoms in A), with or without a prodromal or residual phase, as defined below.
  Prodromal phase: A clear deterioration in functioning before the active phase of the disturbance that is not due to a disturbance in mood or to a Psychoactive Substance Use Disorder and that involves at least two of the symptoms listed below.
  Residual phase: Following the active phase of the disturbance, persistence of at least two of the symptoms noted below, these not being due to a disturbance in mood or to a Psychoactive Substance Use Disorder.
  Prodromal or Residual Symptoms:
  (1) marked social isolation or withdrawal
  (2) marked impairment in role functioning as wage-earner, student, or homemaker
  (3) markedly peculiar behavior (e.g., collecting garbage, talking to self in public, hoarding food)
  (4) marked impairment in personal hygiene and grooming
  (5) blunted or inappropriate affect
  (6) digressive, vague, overelaborate, or circumstantial speech, or poverty of speech, or poverty of content of speech
  (7) odd beliefs or magical thinking, influencing behavior and inconsistent with cultural norms, e.g., superstitiousness, belief in clairvoyance, telepathy, "sixth sense," "others can feel my feelings," overvalued ideas, ideas of reference
  (8) unusual perceptual experiences, e.g., recurrent illusions, sensing the presence of a force or person not actually present
  (9) marked lack of initiative, interests, or energy
  Examples: Six months of prodromal symptoms with one week of symptoms from A; no prodromal symptoms with six months of symptoms from A; no prodromal symptoms with one week of symptoms from A and six months of residual symptoms.
E. It cannot be established that an organic factor initiated and maintained the disturbance.
F. If there is a history of Autistic Disorder, the additional diagnosis of Schizophrenia is made only if prominent delusions or hallucinations are also present.

(American Psychiatric Association, 1987)

pression (Lewis, 1971). Cullen used it as equivalent to vesania, but gradually it assumed the meaning of a primary delusional condition in a setting of clear consciousness. Kraepelin initially classified paranoia as a separate entity from dementia praecox. It represented the insidious development of a delusional system in the presence of an intact personality. He used the term *paraphrenia* to refer to those who have a paranoid illness developing later in life than dementia praecox. Lewis (1971), after a careful consideration of the world literature, gave the following definition: "A paranoid syndrome is one in which there are delusions of self reference which may be concerned with persecution, grandeur, litigation, jealousy, love, envy, hate, honour, or the supernatural, and which cannot be immediately derived from a prevailing morbid mood such as mania or depression" (p. 11).

He felt that the adjective *paranoid* could be applied to a personality disorder with similar features, except that dominant ideas should replace delusions.

The ICD-9 has several categories of paranoid states, and refers to paranoia as a rare chronic psychosis. The DSM-III-R has delusional disorders characterised by persistent nonbizarre delusions not attributable to any other mental disorder. Again there is an exclusion from making this diagnosis if there is an organic factor involved. The term *nonbizarre* refers to ideas pertaining to ordinary life; for example, being followed or poisoned, as opposed to the more florid manifestations of the schizophrenic.

ORGANIC MENTAL SYNDROMES

In DSM-III-R the distinction is made between organic mental syndromes and organic mental disorders. The term *syndrome* has no reference to aetiology, whereas the term *disorder* is used where aetiology is known or can be presumed. Any underlying condition is listed in Axis III.

The organic mental syndromes are given in Table 3.9. The organic mental disor-

---

TABLE 3.9. *Organic Mental Syndromes from DSM-III-R*

The Organic Mental Syndromes can be grouped into six categories:
  (1) **Delirium and Dementia,** in which cognitive impairment is relatively global;
  (2) **Amnestic Syndrome and Organic Hallucinosis,** in which relatively selective areas of cognition are impaired;
  (3) **Organic Delusional Syndrome, Organic Mood Syndrome, and Organic Anxiety Syndrome,** which have features resembling Schizophrenic, Mood, and Anxiety Disorders;
  (4) **Organic Personality Syndrome,** in which the personality is affected;
  (5) **Intoxication and Withdrawal,** in which the disorder is associated with ingestion of or reduction in use of a psychoactive substance and does not meet the criteria for any of the previous syndromes (Strictly speaking, these two Organic Mental Syndromes are etiologically rather than descriptively defined.);
  (6) **Organic Mental Syndrome Not Otherwise Specified,** which constitutes a residual category for any other Organic Mental Syndrome not classifiable as one of the previous syndromes.

(American Psychiatric Association, 1987)

TABLE 3.10A. *Diagnostic Criteria for Organic Delusional Syndrome from DSM-III-R*

A. Prominent delusions.
B. There is evidence from the history, physical examination, or laboratory of a specific organic factor (or factors) judged to be etiologically related to disturbance.
C. Not occurring exclusively during the course of Delirium.

(American Psychiatric Association, 1987)

ders subdivide into three categories: dementia, substance abuse, and the organic mental disorders whose aetiology is an Axis III condition.

This classification is at once both confusing and confused. However, more problematic is the use of the term *organic*, setting it up against, for example, other psychoses where organic factors must be presumed to be absent. An earlier terminological confusion, that between functional and organic, has been perpetuated.

The term *functional* was originally introduced to refer to alteration of brain function, as opposed to structure (Trimble, 1982). In the nineteenth century, the phrenologists, especially, were responsible for shifting its use to a psychological one; namely, categorising mental functions and associating them with discrete brain regions. "Functional" gradually became synonymous with the mental as opposed to the physical, being contrasted with "organic." The latter was clearly related to the identification of structural cerebral changes, and neurology as a discipline was founded upon identification of such change in vivo in association with symptoms. "Functional" became associated with "psychiatric", but soon lost all meaning, being used variously as an expression of clinical ignorance, a means to patient discharge from hospital, or as a polite epithet for malingering.

Since the 1950s and the clear understanding of the role of neurotransmitters in modulating neuronal activity, "functional" has again become used in the sense of referring to brain function, and to consideration as to how this is influenced by

TABLE 3.10B. *Diagnostic Criteria for Organic Personality Syndrome DSM-III-R*

A. A persistent personality disturbance, either lifelong or representing a change or accentuation of a previously characteristic trait, involving at least one of the following:
   (1) affective instability, e.g., marked shifts from normal mood to depression, irritability, or anxiety
   (2) recurrent outbursts of aggression or rage that are grossly out of proportion to any precipitating psychosocial stressors
   (3) markedly impaired social judgment, e.g., sexual indiscretions
   (4) marked apathy and indifference
   (5) suspiciousness or paranoid ideation
B. There is evidence from the history, physical examination, or laboratory tests of a specific organic factor (or factors) judged to be etiologically related to the disturbance.
C. This diagnosis is not given to a child or adolescent if the clinical picture is limited to the features that characterize Attention-deficit Hyperactivity Disorder (see p. 50).
D. Not occurring exclusively during the course of Delirium, and does not meet the criteria for Dementia.
Specify explosive type if outbursts of aggression or rage are the predominant feature.

(American Psychiatric Association, 1987)

disease. Organic change; that is, structural neuronal damage, always leads to functional change, although the latter may occur in the absence of the former through neurophysiological and neurochemical alterations. However, it is obvious that such use of the term *functional* implies organic, that is, corporeal, change; further, at the microstructural level, for example, at the receptor, the distinction becomes very blurred.

Organic and functional are thus complementary rather than polar opposites. Appreciation of this is fundamental to understanding the pathogenesis of the symptoms of many CNS disorders, from the structural damage caused by a stroke to the largely functional changes associated with a major affective disorder. Many disorders are associated with maximal functional change in the presence of variable organic pathology, and schizophrenia and epilepsy are two examples. In some cases this may reflect on the inadequacy of detecting alterations of structure, since the more refined our techniques for assessing the brain in vivo and at postmortem examination, the more the functional disorders have become associated with underlying structural abnormalities.

ICD-9 is of little further help, having a category "other organic psychotic conditions (chronic)," covering a variety of conditions from the dementia of Huntington's chorea to epileptic psychosis. The proposed ICD-10 is somewhat improved, having under the category "Organic and Symptomatic Mental Disorders" a subgroup of "other psychotic, emotional and mood disorders secondary to brain damage or physical disease."

DSM-III-R has the headings: "Organic Delusional Syndrome," "Organic Hallucinosis," "Organic Mood Disorder," "Organic Anxiety Syndrome," and "Organic Personality Syndrome [or disorder!]." The criteria for some of these are given in Table 3.10. These are inadequate to cover the epileptic psychoses. It will be argued that the schizophrenia-like psychosis of epilepsy has distinguishing features which necessitate a separate designation, as do some of the personality disorders of epilepsy.

4

The Limbic System and Related Anatomical Connections

Developments in understanding brain structure and interrelationships between different brain regions have expanded greatly in the past few years. This progress has stemmed from a renewed interest in brain-behaviour relationships from psychiatrists, neurologists, and behavioural psychologists, and from the advancement of techniques from staining neurones and fibre tracts. The latter endeavour has essentially resulted in an entirely new map of the brain emerging, and a multitude of neuronal interrelationships are now known to exist forming a basis for speculation about and correlation with behavioural repertoires.

In this chapter the essential features of the neuroanatomy and neurochemistry of the limbic system are presented, as well as an introduction to the pathology of epilepsy. It is already apparent from earlier chapters that the most important and, as will be shown later, the most demonstrable relationships between epilepsy and psychopathology are those between limbic epilepsy, personality disorders, and psychoses. It is not intended to imply that all of the behavioural problems encountered in epilepsy can be explained by an understanding of the limbic system; neither is it to be inferred that the limbic system operates in isolation, dissociated from other areas of the brain.

THE LIMBIC SYSTEM

Willis (1622–1675), in his *Cerebri Anatome*, referred to an area of the brain around the brainstem as the *cerebri limbus*, and Broca (1824–1880) (1878) defined the comparative anatomy of a region of cerebral cortex which included the hippocampus and the parahippocampal, subcallosal, and cingulate gyri as *le grand lobe limbique*. Although primarily an anatomical definition, he noted the close connection of this to the olfactory apparatus, which led to the adoption of the term *rhinencephalon*. This name and the association with olfaction, remained until the middle of this century when the concept of the limbic system was elaborated in the writings of Papez (1937), Yakovlev (1948), and MacLean (1970). Papez, in his 1937 paper "A proposed mechanism of emotion," laid down a neurological substrate for emotion, and defined the so-called Papez circuit. This was composed of the neuronal elements shown in Fig. 4.1. He contrasted the activities of the medial cortex (with the hippocampus and cingulate cortex participating in hypothalamic activity) with the general sensory activities of the lateral cortex linking with the dorsal thalamus.

MacLean emphasised how the limbic system, which has grown considerably in mammals, has a common structure. The limbic system is divided into two: the archicortex, so called because it is the first type of cortex to differentiate; and the mesocortex, which is intermediate in structure between archicortex and neocortex. These nonneocortical areas of cortex are collectively referred to as allocortex. In man, on account of the migration of the temporal lobes posteriorly, inferiorly, and then anteriorly, and the large increase in size of the corpus callosum, much of the archicortex lies folded and buried in the medial temporal lobe in the hippocampus. In contrast to the neocortex, the limbic cortex has rich connections with the hypothalamus and the central grey regions of the midbrain. Further, limbic system structures all show a low seizure threshold and seizure activity can be confined within them. Stevens (1986) has argued that the existence of a group of structures in the brain with a low seizure threshold would be a threat to survival unless nature had taken the precaution to prevent propagation of seizure discharges beyond such circuits to brain areas modulating motor, sensory, and cognitive function. The more so

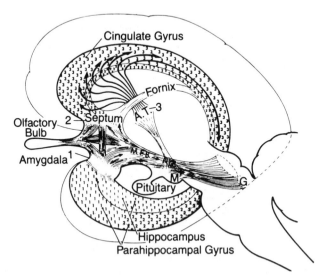

FIG. 4.1. An anatomic framework for considering functions of three main subdivisions of limbic system. Cortical sectors of three divisions are indicated by overlying small numerals, while associated nuclear groups are correspondingly identified by large numerals. A.T. indicates anterior thalamic nuclei; G, tegmental nuclei of Gudden; HYP, hypothalamus; M, mammillary bodies; M.F.B., medial forebrain bundle. (From MacLean, 1970, with permission.)

since she commented that rapid synchronous firing of neurones in discrete nuclei of the limbic system, brainstem, and hypothalamus is associated with many physiological functions such as parturition, milk ejection, or even orgasm in man. Such "microseizures" are thus a part of a neuronal signal system and are not pathological. She argues for a steep voltage gradient provided by extensive inhibitory networks restricting propagation and suggests that this wall of "inhibition" is maintained by the action of several inhibitory transmitters, including gamma-aminobutyric acid (GABA), dopamine, and noradrenaline.

The structures that comprise the limbic system vary from author to author. Mac-Lean (1970) stressed the common link to the hypothalamus, and included the hippocampal formation, the amygdala, the insula, the septum, the habenula, some thalamic nuclei, parts of the basal ganglia, and the gyrus fornicatus (the cingulate gyrus, retrosplenial cortex, and parahippocampal gyrus). Further included are the large interconnecting pathways such as the medial forebrain bundle (MFB), stria terminalis, fornix, and the mammillothalamic tract (see Fig. 4.1 and Table 4.1).

Nauta and Domesick (1982) have discussed the inclusion of other structures. These include posterior orbitofrontal cortex and temporal pole, which project to the amygdala and hippocampus, and some subcortical structures linked by reciprocal pathways. The latter are such structures as the nucleus accumbens, a striatal element, and midbrain structures such as the ventral tegmental area (VTA) and the interpeduncular nucleus. The inclusion of the latter has led to the designation of a midbrain limbic area, the mesolimbic system. These latter connections, unappreciated until recently, also include several nuclei, which are located at the junction of the midbrain and the pons, that have extensive limbic connections but which also receive visceral input from vagal and glossopharyngeal afferents via the solitary nucleus. These include the dorsal and ventral tegmental nuclei of Gudden, the parabrachial nuclei, the raphe nuclei, and the locus ceruleus.

TABLE 4.1. *A List of Limbic System Structures*

Gyri	Nuclei	Pathways
Subcallosal G	Amygdaloid N	Fornix
Cingulate G	Septal N	Mammillothalamic tract
Parahippocampal G	Hypothalamic N	Mammillotegmental tract
Hippocampal	Epithalamic N	Stria terminalis
formation	Anterior thalamic N	Stria medullaris
Dentate G	Mammillary bodies	Cingulum
Indusium griseum	Habenula	Anterior commissure
Subiculum	Raphe N	Medial forebrain bundle
Entorhinal area	Ventral tegmental	Lateral and medial longitudinal striae
Prepiriform cortex	area	Dorsal longitudinal fasciculus
Olfactory tubercle	Dorsal tegmental N	
	Superior central N	

(Trimble, 1981)

Amygdala

This is found in the depth of the medial temporal lobe. It is medial to the inferior horn of the lateral ventricle. Various subdivisions of its nuclei have been suggested, most recognising a lateral and a medial group. The basal nucleus has a high acetylcholine (ACH) content, and projects to the basal nucleus of Meynert, which (see below) provides a widespread cholinergic influence on the cerebral cortex.

The main afferent and efferent pathways traverse the stria terminalis and the ventral amygdalofugal pathway. The latter is a longitudinal association bundle linking to the ventral striatum (see below) and the medial frontal cortex. There is also a medial amygdalohypothalamic bundle going to the lateral hypothalamus and via the MFB to the brainstem, the uncinate fasciculus (which projects to the frontal cortex), and the diagonal band of Broca to the septal and hypothalamic regions.

The connections to the brainstem come almost exclusively from the central nucleus of the medial group, the fibres ending in several structures that serve autonomic and visceral functions. These include the catecholamine and serotonin brainstem nuclei, the VTA and the substantia nigra, the central grey nuclei, the dorsal nucleus of the vagus, and the nucleus of the solitary tract.

The basolateral area has cortical and ventral striatal links, being reciprocally connected with the adjacent temporal cortex and providing afferents to motor and premotor cortices. It is also reciprocally related to the thalamus. The basomedial group, with its connections to the hypothalamus, forms a continuum with the bed nucleus of the stria terminalis in the forebrain, the substantia innominata, and the centromedial amygdala, referred to as the "extended amygdala" (Alheid and Heimer, 1988). In the cortex, amygdaloid fibres are found in the orbital and medial frontal lobes, the rostral cingulate gyrus, and most of the temporal lobe (Price, 1981).

The connections of the amygdala to the hippocampus are primarily via the entorhinal cortex (see below), which is a major source of hippocampal afferents. Those to the hypothalamus may influence the control of pituitary hormone release, especially the projections to the ventromedial nucleus, which itself projects to the arcuate nucleus. Some of these connections are shown diagrammatically in Fig. 4.2.

GABA is an important inhibitory transmitter in the amygdala; other neurotransmitters identified in it include ACh, histamine, dopamine (especially in the basolateral and central nuclei), noradrenaline, serotonin; and the peptides such as substance P, metencephalin, somatostatin (Ben-Ari, 1981), vasoactive intestinal peptide (VIP), and neurotensin.

Hippocampus

The hippocampal structures are closely linked to the septal nuclei, sometimes referred to as the septohippocampal system. The expansion and development of the

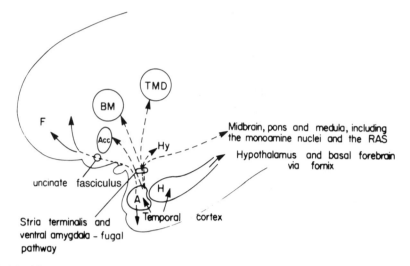

FIG. 4.2. Afferent and efferent projections (*arrows*) of the amygdala. Note the extensive inputs from the temporal cortex and widespread influence on a number of important areas from the frontal cortex to the brainstem. A = amygdala; Acc = nucleus accumbens; BM = basal nucleus of Meynert; F = frontal and cingulate areas; H = hippocampus; Hy = hypothalamus; TMD = mediodorsal nucleus of thalamus; RAS = Reticular Activation System.

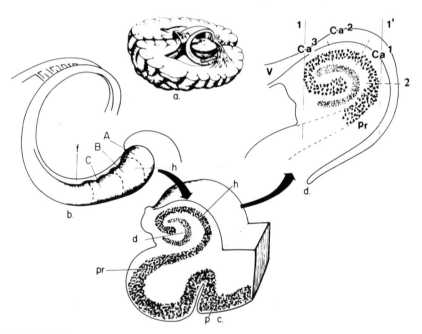

FIG. 4.3. The hippocampus and its structure: a.) horizontally cut hemispheres showing location of hippocampus; b.) enlargement of hippocampus and fornix showing location of (A) anterior, (B) middle, and (C) hippocampal segments; c.) enlargement of single hippocampal segment showing (h) position of hippocampus, (d) fascia dentate, (pr) prosubiculum, and (p) parahippocampal gyrus; d.) diagram illustrating locations of subdivisions of cornu ammonis, CA-1, CA-2, and CA-3 between reference lines 1, 1', and 2'; (V) is lateral ventricle. (From Kovelman and Scheibel, 1984, with permission.)

human brain leads these two structures to be far separated, but in lower animals they are closely linked. Gray (1982) likens this to a pair of joined bananas, where they join being the septal area, and progression from anterior to posterior is accompanied by the structures spreading laterally as they descend into the temporal lobes. The main fibre systems connecting the two are the fimbria and the fornix, and the two hippocampi are interconnected by the hippocampal commissures.

The structure of the hippocampus displays a constant architectural pattern of, as Ramón y Cajal (1955) observed, a "curvilinear palisade of pyramidal cells." Three main divisions are recognised. These are the fascia dentata, Ammon's horn, and the subiculum. This is shown in Fig. 4.3.

The fascia dentata consists of a compact layer of granular cells that form a U-shape and embraces the pyramidal cells of Ammon's horn. The latter is subdivided into four areas, CA1–CA4, in the Lorente de Nó notation (Fig. 4.4). The CA4 and CA3 regions lie embraced by the dentate cells and adjacent to the fimbria, respectively. Here the pyramidal cells are larger than those of CA1 and CA2, and give off the Schaffer collaterals. The prosubiculum lies beyond the CA1 cells, and

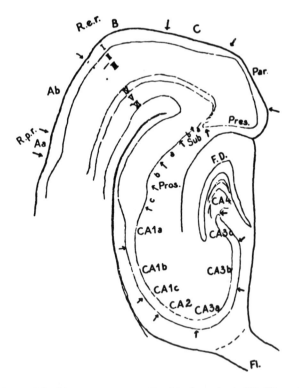

FIG. 4.4. Anatomy of the hippocampus as outlined by Lorente de Nó. (Reproduced with permission.)

here the pyramidal cell dendrites lose their radiate appearance. The subiculum contains perforating fibres to and from the entorhinal cortex. It has a transitional structure, and the neat arrangement seen in Ammon's horn breaks down as it merges with six layered neocortices.

It should be noted that the CA1 area in man is particularly prominent and susceptible to damage by anoxia (an alternative name is Sommer's sector), and afferents from the septum largely terminate in CA3 and CA4, as do the commissural connections from the opposite hippocampus. The laminar organisation of the hippocampus is derived from its regular cell layers, notably the pyramidal cells, granular cells, and the interneuronal inhibitory basket cells. Essentially, the circuit of information flow from the neocortex is from the parahippocampal gyrus and entorhinal cortex via the perforant path to the dentate gyrus, then from the CA3 to the CA1 areas and the subiculum. The latter feeds into the fornix and back to the parahippocampal gyrus and neocortex. As noted, interoceptive information flows via the fornix to and from the hypothalamus, septum, the thalamus (notably the mammillary bodies), and the midbrain limbic areas. The CA3 area is rich in connectivity and there is a 5% chance of any CA3 neurone synapsing with another. It forms an excellent funnel for diverse exteroceptive and interoceptive information to coalesce and is functionally related to memory.

The main neurotransmitter associated with inhibition in the hippocampus is GABA, but the structure receives dopaminergic, serotoninergic and noradrenergic afferents. Peptides such as VIP, cholecystokinin (CCK), neurotensin, somatostatin, substance P, and metencephalin have been identified in the hippocampus (Roberts et al., 1984).

The Parahippocampal Gyrus

This structure is of central importance in the limbic system. It is adjacent to and continuous with the hippocampus and includes, progressing caudally, the piriform, entorhinal, and parahippocampal cortices. In that it has only poorly defined cortical layers, it has been referred to as schizocortex (split cortex). In Brodmann's system, the entorhinal cortex is represented by area 28 (Fig. 4.5). It has extensive projections to the hippocampal formation via the perforant pathway and, most importantly, cortical afferents from many cortical sites. Thus, the association cortices project to this region, providing limbic system input of visual, auditory, and somatic information. Further, as noted, the amygdala, with its strong hypothalamic connections, projects to the entorhinal area such that the hippocampus receives, via the parahippocampal gyrus, multimodal sensory information derived from the external and internal world.

The subiculum also projects to the parahippocampal gyrus, and the latter, in turn, has widespread limbic and association cortical projections to frontal, parietal, temporal, and occipital lobes (Fig. 4.6) (Van Hoesen, 1982).

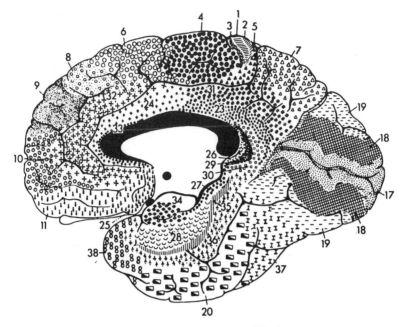

FIG. 4.5. The anatomical areas of Brodmann.

The Septal Area

The septal nuclei are situated below the corpus callosum, ventrally bounded by the olfactory tubercle and the nucleus accumbens. The lateral boundary is made by the lateral ventricle, and the caudal boundary by the third ventricle and hypothalamus (Fig. 4.7). In man, the dorsal part is elongated by the development of the corpus callosum to form the septum pellucidum which forms a glial and fibre attachment to the corpus callosum.

The septal area is usually subdivided into medial and lateral groups. The medial septal area is further divided into the medial septal nucleus and the nucleus of the diagonal band of Broca, both of which contain ACh and project to the hippocampus and the entorhinal cortex via the fimbria and fornix. The lateral nuclei receive hippocampal afferents, mainly from CA3 and the subiculum. Since the lateral and medial septal nuclei interconnect, a functional circuit is derived as follows:

HIPPOCAMPUS → LATERAL SEPTUM → MEDIAL SEPTUM →
HIPPOCAMPUS

Also shown in Fig. 4.7 is the bed nucleus of the stria terminalis (which receives amygdala projections) and the substantia innominata (part of the extended amygdala).

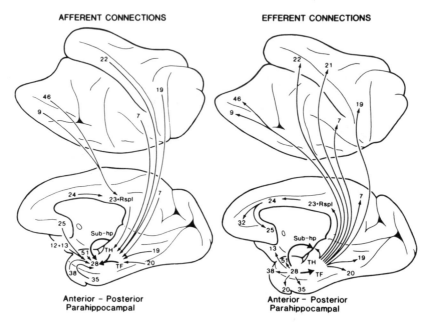

FIG. 4.6. Summary of cortical afferent and efferent connections of the rhesus monkey parahippocampal gyrus shown on lateral (inverted) and medial views of the cerebral hemisphere. With regard to afferent connections, the projections from areas 12, 13, 23, 24, 25, 35, 38, 51, retrosplenial cortex (Rspl), subiculumhippocampus (Sub-hp) and posterior parahippocampal area (TF, TH) represent intrinsic pathways within the limbic lobe that converge on area 28, the entorhinal cortex. The area 51 projections would be expected to carry olfactory input. Projections from areas 19 and 20 to areas TF, TH are visual association projections; those from area 22 are auditory association projections; those from area 7 are visuo-somatic projections and those from areas 9 and 46 are frontal association projections. Multimodal projections from the cortex in the superior temporal sulcus are not shown. The heavy-lined arrows from Sub-hp and TF, TH to area 28 denote that there are two of the heaviest sources of input to this cortex. With regard to efferent or output projections, note that there is a nearly exact reciprocation of the input pathways. The heavy line from areas 28 to Sub-hp represents the perforant pathway. (From Jones and Powell, 1970, with permission.)

The septal area receives rich monoamine projections, especially dopamine, from the ventral tegmental area via the MFB. VIP, CCK, somatostatin, metenkephalin, neurotensin, and substance P are all found in the septum.

The Cingulate Gyrus

This runs ventral to the corpus callosum, following a C-shaped curve as it progresses posteriorly. The anterior cingulate region is the area outlined by Brodmann as areas 24, 25, and 32. The posterior and retrosplenial areas are regions 23, 26, 29, and 30 (see Fig. 4.5.), and here the cingulate gyrus becomes narrow and continuous with the lingual gyrus, a dorsal extension of the parahippocampal gyrus. The cingu-

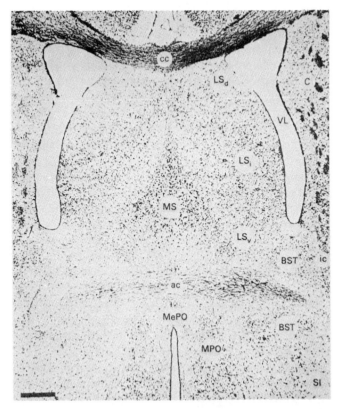

FIG. 4.7. The septal area. BST = bed nucleus of stria terminalis; C = caudate nucleus; LS = lateral septal nuclei; MePO = median preoptic nucleus; MPO = medial preoptic nucleus; MS = medial septal nucleus; VL = lateral ventricle; ac = anterior commissure; SI = substantia innominata; cc = corpus callosum. (From Swanson, 1978. Reproduced with permission.)

late cortex is continuous with the frontal cortex anteriorly, is rich in dopamine fibres, and contains CCK and opiate receptors.

Hypothalamus

The hypothalamus, positioned dorsal to the pituitary gland, is a site of convergence for much limbic system activity. It is the main subcortical projection site of much older cortex, and has no direct neocortical input. Posterior to it are the mammillary bodies, and anteriorly are the optic chiasm and the preoptic area. The descending fornix divides the hypothalamus into medial and lateral areas. The medial border of the medial hypothalamus is formed by the third ventricle, and several nuclear groups are defined. The suprachiasmatic nucleus is thought to be a regulator of rhythmic activity, a sort of "biological clock." The axons of neurones from the supraoptic and paraventricular nuclei are neurosecretory fibres travelling mainly to the posterior pituitary gland.

The lateral area contains many fibres of passage of the monoamine brainstem and midbrain nuclei travelling with the MFB, but the fornix, stria terminalis, and the mammillothalamic tract connect anteriorly; the mammillotegmental tract and dorsal longitudinal fasciculus posteriorly.

Several of the hypothalamic nuclei secrete neuropeptides, some of which are releasing hormones. Thus, these are released into the hypophysial-portal blood vessels which carry them to the anterior pituitary, where they stimulate or inhibit various pituitary hormones.

The hypothalamus contains many peptide and monoamine neuromodulators including substance P, neurotensin, angiotensin, leu- and metencephalin, beta-endorphin, VIP, CCK, dopamine, noradrenaline, ACh, and serotonin. Dopamine is a prolactin inhibitory factor.

ASCENDING AND DESCENDING LIMBIC SYSTEM CONNECTIONS

The "limbic forebrain-midbrain circuit" exists, which unites the monoamine- and peptide-rich zones of the midbrain with the rostral structures such as the hippocampus, amygdala, and the septal area. A limbic midbrain area has been defined in the paramedian zone of the mesencephalon (Nauta and Domesick, 1982). The main connecting structure is the MFB (Fig. 4.8), a poorly defined fibre system with a loose arrangement characteristic of brainstem reticular formation. It receives contributions from such structures as the septal nuclei, hypothalamus, olfactory tubercle, substantia innominata, nucleus accumbens, amygdala, bed nucleus of stria terminalis, and the orbitofrontal cortex. Caudally it projects to the VTA, the interpeduncular nucleus, the raphe nuclei, the locus ceruleus, and the midbrain reticular formation. It further descends to autonomic and spinal nuclei, including the solitary nucleus.

The ascending components of this limbic forebrain-midbrain circuit arise from important nuclei such as those found in the VTA, the raphe nuclei, the locus ceruleus, and other tegmental nuclei mentioned above. The VTA occupies the basomedial midbrain, dorsal to the substantia nigra, and is continuous rostrally with the lateral hypothalamus. It borders on the ventral periaqueductal grey substance, the dorsal raphe nuclei, and other nuclei of the limbic midbrain. The main ascending connections (Fig. 4.9) are from the dopamine-rich cells that innervate the nucleus accumbens, olfactory tubercle, amygdala, entorhinal area, frontocingulate cortex, and septal area.

The catecholamine nuclei are found in relatively discrete areas of the brainstem, and their fibre paths were first identified using fluorescent histochemical techniques. From the substantia nigra and the VTA arise the majority of dopamine neurones that project to the limbic system (the so-called mesolimbic system) and striatum. The noradrenergic fibres derive largely from the locus ceruleus. In a simi-

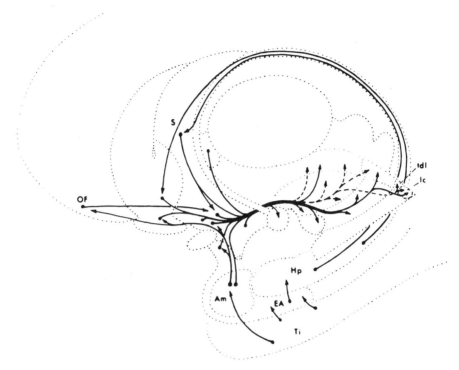

FIG. 4.8. The main connecting pathways of the medial forebrain bundle (MFB). OF = orbitofrontal cortex; lc = locus ceruleus; S = septum; tdl = nucleus tegmenti dorsalis lateralis; EA = entorhinal area; Am = amygdala; Ti = temporal cortex; Hp = hippocampus. (From Nauta and Domesick, 1982, with permission.)

lar fashion, the serotonergic neurones are confined virtually to the brainstem raphe nuclei.

The termination areas for the dopaminergic projections are quite restricted, in contrast to those from the ascending catecholamine neurones which distribute widely, exerting a tonic modulatory influence on many cortical neurones. Serotonin distribution is intermediate, being more extensive than dopamine, projecting to the hippocampus and amygdala, parahippocampal gyrus, habenula, thalamus, and neocortex.

THE BASAL GANGLIA

This term usually refers to the caudate nucleus, putamen, and globus pallidus, although it may include such structures as the subthalamic nucleus and the substantia nigra. Although the amygdala is closely related developmentally, it is considered as part of the limbic system. The striatum refers to the caudate nucleus and putamen, divided as they are by the internal capsule. The caudate nucleus is a large

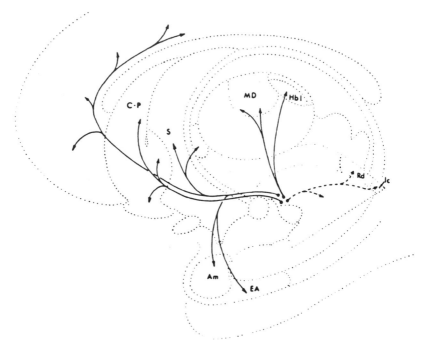

FIG. 4.9. Ascending connections from the dopamine limbic midbrain. C-P = caudate putamen; S = septal area; MD = mediodorsal nucleus of thalamus; Hbl = habenula; Am = amygdala; EA = entorhinal area; Rd = dorsal raphe nucleus; lc = locus ceruleus. (From Nauta and Domesick, 1982, with permission.)

curved nucleus which adheres throughout its length to the lateral ventricles, anteriorly being continuous with the putamen.

The afferent connections to the striatum are from the cerebral cortex, thalamic nuclei, the substantia nigra, the amygdala and the raphe nucleus. The most investigated is the dopamine-rich nigrostriatal projection, mainly on account of its obvious association with Parkinson's disease.

The corticostriate connections come from nearly all regions of the neocortex, projecting onto the striatum topographically. Motor cortex (Brodmann's area 4, see Fig. 4.5) and somatosensory cortex (areas 3,1, and 2) project to the putamen, while prefrontal and other association cortices preferentially project to the caudate nucleus. The thalamostriate connections come from nonspecific cell groups.

Efferent connections are via the globus pallidus, some fibres traversing this and establishing a striatonigral connection. The striatopallidal projection is rich in enkephalin, and the striatonigral in substance P. Other peptides and neurotransmitters related to these structures include the GABA-dominated striatonigral link; the presence of enkephalin-like substance P and CCK immunoreactivity in the substantia nigra; and the presence of ACH, enkephalin, neurotensin, somatostatin, substance

P, and opiate binding in the striatum (Graybiel, 1984). The large corticostriate projection is thought to be glutaminergic.

The efferent connections of the globus pallidus travel through the ansa lenticularis to the subthalamus, thalamus, habenula, and midbrain tegmentum.

THE VENTRAL STRIATUM AND "LIMBIC STRIATUM"

The anatomy of the basal forebrain, that group of ventral structures underneath or at the level of the anterior commissure, and its relationship to behaviour have been reevaluated in recent years. Much attention has focussed on dopamine-rich structures lying ventral and medial to, and associated with, the head of the caudate nucleus. One such structure is the nucleus accumbens. This, together with the closely associated olfactory tubercle and ventromedial parts of the caudatoputamen, has been referred to as the ventral striatum (Heimer et al., 1982). Its caudal boundary with the bed nucleus of the stria terminalis is difficult to establish, but anteriorly it extends into the ventromedial portion of the frontal lobe, and it lies lateral to the septal region (White, 1981).

The ventral striatum has a close anatomical, developmental, and structural relationship to the striatum. Both structures receive a dopaminergic input from VTA and have limbic system connections. In particular, the ventral striatum receives projections from the hippocampus via the fornix, the amygdala, and the frontal cortex, this allocortical input contrasting with the neocortical dorsal striatum connections (Fig. 4.10). Thus, as a generalisation, it can be said that most afferents to the nucleus accumbens come from the limbic system. Others come from the thalamus and hypothalamus. The nucleus accumbens is located at the interface of limbic projections from the hippocampus, amygdala, and cingulate cortex and receives extrapyramidal input from midbrain dopaminergic nuclei.

As fibres leave the nucleus accumbens they project to a rostroventral extension of the globus pallidus, referred to as the ventral pallidum. This region is also called the substantia innominata, an area rich in ACH (it forms part of the basal nucleus of Meynert) and substance P. The ventral pallidum projects to the mediodorsal nucleus of the thalamus, which in turn projects to the prefrontal, limbic, and cingulate cortices (Heimer et al., 1982). Thus the circuit:

LIMBIC CORTEX → VENTRAL STRIATUM → VENTRAL PALLIDUM →
THALAMUS → LIMBIC CORTEX

is a counterpart to the other corticostriate loop in which the dorsal globus pallidus projects to the ventral anterior thalamic nucleus:

NEOCORTEX → STRIATUM → GLOBUS PALLIDUS → THALAMUS →
NEOCORTEX

Substance P, enkephalin, and CCK are found in both ventral striatum and dorsal striatum, while VIP, thyrotropin releasing hormone (TRH), and neurotensin are

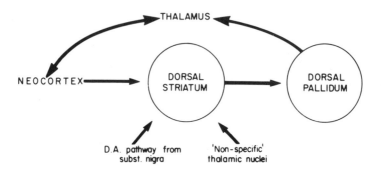

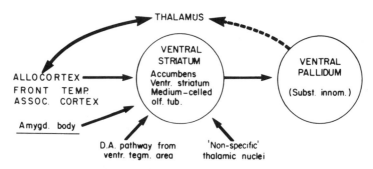

FIG. 4.10. Different connections of the dorsal and ventral striatum. Note the predominant limbic connections with the latter. D.A. = dopamine.

found mainly in the nucleus accumbens. Other peptides located in the nucleus accumbens include somatostatin and melanocyte-stimulating hormone (MSH) (Johannsson and Hokfelt, 1981). There are also high concentrations of ACH, glutamate, and GABA. It is efferent GABAergic fibres from the nucleus accumbens to the ventral pallidum that translate limbic and extrapyramidal information to motor output.

Some of the contrasts between the dorsal striatum and the ventral striatum are shown in Table 4.2.

Nauta has repeatedly emphasised the crosstalk between the limbic system and the basal ganglia (Nauta and Domesick, 1982). These are of obvious importance in understanding links between motor and emotional behaviour (Trimble, 1981), but additionally have relevance as neuroanatomical substrates for the development of psychopathology in epilepsy. In addition to the direct connections between the hippocampus, amygdala, cingulate cortex, and the ventral striatum; the habenula has both limbic and pallidal afferents. Further, indirect links by way of the substantia nigra and raphe nucleus exist. Thus, cells of the substantia nigra are influenced by the descending fibres of the MFB and the fasciculus retroflexus from the habenulae.

TABLE 4.2. *Some Contrasts Between the Dorsal Striatum and Ventral Striatum*

	Dorsal	Ventral
Dopamine projection	Mainly A9 (substantia nigra)	Mainly A10 (VTA)
Cortical afferents	Limbic and neocortical	Limbic
Main efferents	Dorsal pallidum (globus pallidus)	Ventral pallidum

Interestingly, connections in the opposite direction, from striatum to the limbic system, are limited.

Alheid and Heimer (1988) suggest, on histochemical and anatomical grounds, that some components of the nucleus accumbens represent a rostral portion of the extended amygdala, and note that "taken as a whole, the extended amygdala represents a formidable forebrain system which possesses a rather extensive series of connections allowing it to directly influence neuroendocrine, somatomotor and autonomic output" (p. 28).

Further, the extended amygdala can, through its efferents, widely affect cortical function.

One further point of anatomical interest should be made: three limbic projections converge on the anterior ventral component of the striatum; namely, the dopaminergic fibres from the VTA, the amygdala projection, and fibres from the frontal cortex.

THALAMUS AND FRONTAL CORTEX

The thalamus is usually considered to play a key role in the transmission of somatic sensory impulses on their way to the cerebral cortex. It is composed of three main nuclear groups: medial, lateral, and anterior. The ventral posterolateral nucleus conveys medial lemniscal and spinothalamic information to the primary and secondary sensory cortical areas; the basal ganglia afferents project mainly to ventrolateral, ventroanterior, and so-called intralaminar nuclei (located within white matter laminae that transect the thalamus). These thalamic nuclei also receive cerebellar projections; and reciprocal connections with the frontal cortex are made by the ventral, anterior, and mediodorsal nuclei, the anterior nuclei connecting to the cingulate gyrus as part of the Papez circuit.

The reticular formation—that loosely assembled, closely packed network of neurones in the brainstem—activates many thalamic fibres, continuing by relay and direct connection to reach all fields of the cortex, stimulation of which activates the entire forebrain.

The frontal lobes are anatomically represented by those areas of cortex anterior to the central sulcus and, as such, embrace the main cortical representations for the control of motor behaviour. The term *prefrontal cortex* designates the most anterior pole, an area sometimes referred to as the frontal granular cortex, or the frontal association cortex. This is represented by Brodmann's areas 8, 9, 10, 11, 12, 44, 45, 46, and 47 (see Fig. 4.5). One definition of the prefrontal cortex is that region which receives projections from the mediodorsal thalamic nucleus (Fuster, 1980). These are topographically organised such that the medial part of the nucleus projects to the medial and orbitofrontal cortices; the lateral part to the lateral and dorsal cortices. The medial thalamic area receives afferents from the mesencephalic reticular formation and the amygdala, entorhinal cortex, and inferior temporal cortex, whereas the lateral nuclear area has only afferents from the prefrontal cortex (Fuster, 1980).

Other important prefrontal connections are made by the mesocortical dopamine projections from VTA. Further links are to the hypothalamus, the cingulate gyrus, the amygdala, the hippocampus, and the retrosplenial and entorhinal cortices. On the basis of primate data, Nauta (1964) suggested that the orbital frontal cortex made connections with the amygdala and related subcortical structures, whereas the dorsal cortex links more to the hippocampus and parahippocampal gyrus. Certainly there seems to be a circuit comparable to the Papez circuits formed by the amygdala instead of by the hippocampus, thus:

AMYGDALA → THALAMUS (MEDIAL DORSAL N.) → ORBITOFRONTAL CORTEX → INFERIOR TEMPORAL CORTEX → AMYGDALA

In the same way that sensory information from primary sensory cortex, after passing to adjacent secondary areas, cascades to the anterior temporal areas (Jones and Powell, 1970), the prefrontal cortex also is a projection area for somatic, auditory, and sensory information from other cortical areas. The prefrontal cortex is the only neocortical area to receive projections from the visceral nuclei.

The prefrontal cortex projects to, but does not receive afferents from, the striatum. A final point is that the area of the prefrontal cortex that receives the dominant dorsomedial nucleus projection overlaps that from the dopaminergic VTA.

BRAIN STRUCTURE, FUNCTION, AND BEHAVIOUR

The anatomy and connectivity of the limbic system has been defined because many patients with epilepsy have pathology in defined limbic sites (see below) and, as already noted, one form of localisation-related epilepsy may properly be designated as limbic. It is important, in relation to the theme of limbic (especially epileptic-related) behaviour disturbances, to consider some behavioural associations of the limbic system as derived from studies in animals and man. As with the neuroanatomical section, this is a selected review emphasising areas of relevance for epileptic behaviour disturbance.

MacLean (1958, 1990) has repeatedly emphasised the three main subdivisions of the limbic system. These are the amygdala, septal, and thalamocingulate components (see Fig. 4.1). The frontotemporal pole (amygdalar) of the limbic system is primarily concerned with self-preservation, and stimulation leads to two main types of responses. These are licking, chewing and other oral activity; and sniffing, searching, and anger. In contrast, the cingulate gyrus and septum relate to preservation of the species as seen in such activities as grooming and sexual activity. Further, MacLean has emphasised a triad of behaviours; namely, nursing, play, and the isolation call, which are basic for mammalian family life. He relates the growth of limbic system size with the development of such social bonding behaviour as seen in mammals. Of major significance is the comparative anatomical fact that there is no counterpart of the thalamocingulate division of the limbic circuitry outside the mammals. Ablation of the cingulate gyrus leads to a deficit in maternal behaviour and play, and stimulation of the anterior cortex leads to vocalisations.

One of the significant observations of brain-behaviour relationships was that defined by Klüver and Bucy (1939) following the placement of bilateral lesions in the temporal lobes of monkeys. As a consequence the animals became tame, with loss of fear and aggression; hypersexual; demonstrated excessive oral exploration of their environment; and had a visual agnosia. Since the lesions removed the uncus, amygdala, and part of the hippocampus, it was reasonable to assume that the intactness of these structures was a prerequisite for the organisation and control of mood, sexual behaviour, and visual perception (Koella, 1982).

Aggression

The relationship of the amygdala to aggression seems well established, although a reciprocal link with the hypothalamus and frontal cortex seems important. Thus, following on from the Klüver-Bucy experiments, Schriner and Kling (1956) tamed various aggressive feline species with bilateral amygdala lesions, an effect abolished by additional lesions in the ventrolateral hypothalamus. Aggression can be provoked by stimulation of the amygdala, hypothalamus, and the area around the fornix in the diencephalon, and hypothalamic-elicited aggression can be inhibited by stimulation of the ipsilateral frontal cortex (Siegel et al., 1975). Delgado (1966), using implanted intracerebral multilead electrodes to stimulate various regions of the brain in monkeys, also recorded aggressive responses from the ventral posterolateral nucleus of the thalamus, and the central grey area. By studying behaviour in a colony under various conditions of stimulation, he reported that the aggression artificially provoked by stimulation was indistinguishable from spontaneous aggression; Rosvold et al. (1954) have demonstrated how amygdala lesions lead to loss of dominance in a social heirarchy.

Kindling

Adamec, based on studies with kindling, introduced the concept of "limbic permeability." Thus, kindling is an experimental procedure in which small, brief, high-frequency currents are passed across electrodes in an area of brain. At first no effects are seen, but after several trials, usually given on a daily basis, an afterdischarge develops and behaviour changes are seen. As the process continues, eventually the animal will have, in spite of still receiving subthreshold doses, a generalised seizure. The associated changes in brain physiology, as yet unidentified, are long-lasting, and the animal remains susceptible to a seizure on passing the current for a considerable time, possibly for life.

Kindling is best from limbic system structures, but can be obtained from neocortex. It has not been achieved from brainstem or cerebellar stimulation. The underlying neurophysiological explanation for the effect is not known, but it differs from long-term potentiation. Kindling is most easily obtained from the amygdala and piriform cortex (entorhinal and periamygdaloid regions), and although such areas are damaged in the brains of epileptic patients, the role of kindling in epileptogenesis is still unclear. However, interictal spikes are seen early in the process and, in some settings, structural changes, especially to astrocytes, have been observed (Racine, 1989). The phenomenon can be elicited in many different species, but as a generalisation, the higher up in the phylogeny the species, the longer it takes to kindle seizures.

The original literature on kindling emphasised seizures as an endpoint. However, as a biological process it probably has more widespread ramifications. The clinical relevance of kindling is uncertain (Bolwig and Trimble, 1989), but using kindling paradigms, several authors have emphasised the behavioural, in addition to the epileptic, consequences. Adamec and Stark-Adamec (1983) studied defensive behaviour in cats and its modification by partial kindling. By studying two different types of cats, one essentially more timid than the other, traits that emerge early in life and are stable, they were able to note changes in personality consequent on the experimental procedure. The defensiveness was correlated with seizure susceptibility of the amygdala: the more defensive the cat, the lower the afterdischarge threshold and inversely with the seizure susceptibility of the ventral hippocampus. Following the kindling procedure, during which the afterdischarge threshold is reduced in the amygdala, aggressive cats became more defensive, the behaviour changes seeming to be long-lasting. This behaviour change could be blocked by stimulation to the point of afterdischarge from the hippocampus. Limbic permeability, the degree of propagation of seizure activity between limbic system structures and their output fields, was linked with these phenomena, but the behaviour changes were interictal. In other words, the process left marks on the system that were dissociated from the seizures themselves. Their studies further underline the point that kindling results in enhancement of some normal behaviours and attenuation of others. Further, the behavioural outcome of repeated seizures may depend not only on the brain areas stimulated but also on individual behavioural disposition.

Mellanby and colleagues (1989) used the tetanus toxin model to induce seizures in rats with injections into the hippocampus. This provokes seizures for several weeks, but leaves no long-lasting evidence of gross structural damage. The animals demonstrated behaviour changes and memory problems which persisted after the seizures had waned.

One neurochemical consequence of kindling that may have relevance for these behaviour changes has been described by Csernansky et al. (1988). Following amygdala kindling in rats, they reported the animals to be subsensitive to the stereotype-inducing effects of apomorphine. When the animals were given additional stimulations, "superkindled," they became supersensitive to the apomorphine. In both kindled and "superkindled" animals, D-2 receptor binding densities were increased in the corresponding nucleus accumbens to the side kindled. The number of interictal spikes recorded from the stimulating electrode placed at the amygdala was correlated with the changes in apomorphine sensitivity.

Anxiety and the Septohippocampal Link

Gray (1982), on the basis of extensive animal experiments, has postulated the existence of a behavioural inhibition system which modulates anxiety responses. The neural counterpart of this is the septohippocampal circuit, and anxiolytic drugs are thought to act by inhibiting this system. Briefly, lesions of the septal area or the hippocampus lead to a pattern of behaviours similar to that seen after giving anxiolytic drugs, and stimulation of the septal area the opposite. The septohippocampal system, as noted, forms an extensive interconnected neural network and, in Gray's theory, acts with the associated Papez circuit as a comparator, generating predictions about anticipated events and matching them to actual events. Mismatch allows the behavioural inhibition system to dominate, interrupting behaviour and generating a search for alternatives by increased arousal and attention. Gray also discusses the role of ascending monoaminergic systems, especially noradrenaline and serotonin, which again modulate information flow into the hippocampus. In his system, the prefrontal cortex is a comparator for motor programmes, and in man is a route for verbal influences over septohippocampal functions and a possible neurological correlate of obsessive symptoms.

Other functions assigned to the hippocampus, in the light of electrophysiological stimulation and lesion experiments, mainly relate to memory. Although severe memory problems after hippocampal destruction were first defined in man, animal studies produced conflicting data. Several rival theories exist, although all ascribe to the hippocampus a role in higher cognitive function. One suggestion is that it is involved in the construction of spatial maps (O'Keefe and Nadel, 1978), an alternative that it subserves spatial memory. Its precise role in human memory is unclear and relates either to the consolidation of short-term memory or the retrieval of information once remembered.

MacLean (1990) examined the role of the extensive visual input to the posterior hippocampal gyrus, lingual gyrus, and retrosplenial cortex. Thus, in primates there is great expansion of the perilimbic and peristriate cortices in the medial parietal and occipitotemporal regions. Further, the optic radiations make a detour around the lateral ventricle in Meyer's loop, making contributions to posterior hippocampal, parahippocampal, and retrosplenial cortices. MacLean notes how objects in peripheral vision often induce startle and alarm, and such input may be related to the generation of paranoid feelings.

There is substantial evidence that the hippocampus is involved in neuroendocrine regulation. Thus, it binds more corticosterone than any other brain region, a pattern extending along the septotemporal axis. Further, fornix lesions interfere with normally observed corticosteroid responses, and adrenocorticotropic hormone (ACTH) can modify hippocampal responses (Isaacson, 1982).

The septal area also is involved in a variety of behaviours. Lesions here initially lead to irritability and hyperreactivity, and, as with the amygdala, may lead to changes in the threshold for aggression and dominance, depending on the species and the status of the individual. Of most interest, however, has been the observation that stimulation of this area appears to produce reward. Olds and Milner (1954) referred to this and to other sites from which the same effect could be produced as "pleasure centres." The most active sites were along the path of the MFB, and are related to dopaminergic and/or noradrenergic activity. It has been suggested that this reward system may play a role in memory consolidation (Routtenberg, 1979). Pleasurable responses are obtained in humans from septal stimulation, and spike and slow-wave discharges are recorded there during orgasm (Heath, 1972).

Sexual Behaviour

The changes in sexual activity first seen with the Klüver-Bucy syndrome were confirmed in other species, and the amygdala seems to be important. The hypersexuality induced by amygdala destruction can be reversed by septal lesions (Kling et al., 1960), supporting the role of the latter in pleasurable sexual experiences. Penile erection in monkeys can be seen after stimulation of the septum (MacLean and Ploog, 1962), and electrical activity is recorded here in female rabbits and in man with orgasm (Sawyer, 1957; Heath, 1972).

The hypothalamus is clearly involved in sexual behaviour, and lesions in the anterior hypothalamus prevent the hormonal activation of sexual activity (Heimer and Larsson, 1966). There are many steroid binding sites in hypothalamic regions that interact with systemic hormones to modulate behaviour, further interrelated with the influence of monoamine and peptide systems (Herbert, 1984).

Parahippocampal Gyrus

The entorhinal cortex may be viewed as the great gate through which neocortical information reaches the hippocampus and thence other limbic system structures.

There is clear evidence that this region has access to specific sensory and multimodal sensory representations; the links with the amygdala, and hence the hypothalamus and forebrain limbic structures, imply a meeting point for internal and affective data with current and past sensory information. The traffic is both ways, however: from sensory cortices to the limbic system and vice versa, allowing for limbic influences on sensory experiences.

Motion, Emotion, and Motivation

An early attempt to understand the neurological underpinnings of emotional experience was that of Papez, although knowledge of the limbic system has developed substantially since he described his circuit. MacLean (1990) elaborated further on the behavioural relationships derived from comparative and clinical data, emphasising the rise of social bonding relating to increasing limbic system size and complexity. The most significant advances in this field have derived from the anatomical observations of the close links between the limbic system and the basal ganglia, and the role of the latter in motivation. Thus, traditionally the basal ganglia have been viewed as solely related to motor behaviour. However, emotional display involves motor patterns (hence "e-motion"), motor abnormalities are seen in patients with psychiatric illness as a part of the symptomatology (Trimble, 1981), motor disorders are frequently associated with psychopathology (Trimble, 1981), and movement and emotion are linked in common speech (hence "a moving experience"). MacLean (1990) has convincingly argued that in primates, the role of the striatal complex relates additionally to socially communicative displays, especially via the pallidal outflow to the thalamic and midbrain tegmenta.

Nauta (Nauta and Domesick, 1982), as noted, has drawn attention to areas of limbic-striatal integration. Iversen (1984), following observations of alteration of behaviour after stimulation or lesion of either the ventral or dorsal striatum, has emphasised how the former is related to sensorimotor integration of interoceptive information. Damage here leads to impairment of organised motivational behaviour such as exploration of novel environments. In this scheme, the dorsal striatum is seen as initiating neocortically-derived motor behaviour, and the ventral striatum is related to emotional arousal. The nucleus accumbens is one central station in these schemes, with its connections from amygdala, hippocampus, and midbrain limbic areas. It projects to the ventral pallidum, and hence, in association with neocortical and globus pallidus efferents, influences motor behaviour.

The concept of the extended amygdala is also of importance. To quote Alheid and Heimer (1988): "The central amygdala has been shown to be crucially involved in the formation of conditioned responses. One would predict rather dire consequences, therefore, if the functions of the extended amygdala were compromised . . . inappropriate firing of the extended amygdala, as might be the case in clinical and subclinical temporal lobe epilepsy, could potentially result in disorganisation of the feedback to the cognitive and perceptual apparatus of the cortex. In such cases inordinate significance could be attached to inappropriate or trivial external events" (p. 28).

THE PATHOLOGY OF EPILEPSY

One of the earliest studies of the pathology of epilepsy was that of Bouchet and Cazauvieilh (1825). They gave descriptions of patients with both epilepsy and insanity who had pathology in the Cornes d'Ammon, emphasising the common underlying pathology of both disorders. As Berrios (1979) has pointed out, "after Bouchet and Cazauvieilh the view was held in France that no fundamental difference existed between epilepsy and psychosis" (p. 162).

Although a variety of pathological conditions have been associated with epilepsy, ranging from focal cortical dysplasias to tumours and trauma, the form of seizure disorder of relevance here is that of the partial seizure, especially of temporal lobe origin.

Around the time that Hughlings Jackson was noting clinicopathological correlations between lesions in the anteromedial temporal lobe and the reporting by patients of "dreamy states," (Sommer, 1880) others noted the specific sclerosed appearance of Ammon's horn in the brains of epileptic patients. He especially noted changes in the CA1 area, hence the term *Sommer's sector*. However, it remained undecided as to whether such lesions were the cause or an effect of the epilepsy. The classical lesion is nerve cell loss and gliosis in Ammon's horn and the dentate gyrus, so-called mesial (or medial) temporal sclerosis (MTS) (Fig. 4.11).

An early hypothesis of the origin of the sclerosis was that of Earle et al. (1953), who suggested that it was caused by transtentorial herniation of the medial temporal structures at birth. This led to compression of the anterior choroidal and posterior cerebral arteries and subsequent ischaemia of the medial temporal structures. This view was challenged, notably by Falconer and colleagues, following careful pathological examination of brain tissue removed surgically for the treatment of temporal lobe epilepsy (Cavanagh et al., 1958). Their view was that postnatal events, notably anoxia from prolonged febrile convulsions, were the more likely cause. This view was supported by two main lines of evidence, clinical and experimental. Clinically, patients with MTS were more likely to have had an early bout of status epilepticus than those with other lesions (Falconer and Taylor, 1968). Experimentally, status epilepticus in baboons and rats has been shown to lead to ischaemic cell change in hippocampal pyramidal neurones, leading to cell damage. The latter is probably consequent on excessive inward movement of Ca^{2+}, resulting in high intracellular concentrations (Meldrum et al., 1983). Since it is known that patients susceptible to febrile convulsions are more likely to have a family history of similar seizures, the probable sequence of events is seen as the combination of genetic diathesis (leading to the febrile convulsion) and the acquired lesion, the sclerosis, then rendering the individual more liable to have later-onset temporal lobe epilepsy.

MTS is not, however, always found in association with a history of seizures and is usually, in an epileptic brain, associated with other areas of pathology. An exten-

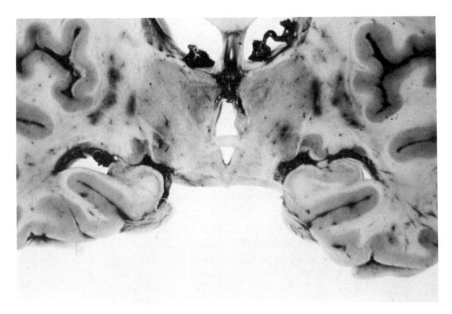

FIG. 4.11. The gross pathology of hippocampal sclerosis in the left hippocampus.

sive pathological series was reported by Margerison and Corsellis (1966). Of 55 cases, hypoxic damage was noted in 44; while it was most frequent in the hippocampus, it was also present in the cerebellum, amygdala, thalamus, and cortex. They noted some cases in which the Sommer sector and dentate gyrus were spared, with cell loss and gliosis in the end folium (CA3 and CA4) and thus used the term *hippocampal sclerosis* to emphasise this variability. The main distinction between those with classical Ammon's horn sclerosis and the patients showing end folium pathology was age of onset of seizures, being 6 years in the former and 16 in the latter.

Scheibel (1991) reported changes maximally in the prosubiculum, CA1 and CA3 areas, with a varying picture in CA4. Dam (1980), using brains from a group of institutionalised patients, noted in contrast that the end folium was maximally affected, in association with a long history of epilepsy.

In the majority of cases the sclerosis is unilateral, although associated cerebellar or cortical changes are bilateral. This unilaterality has not been satisfactorily explained.

Other important pathological lesions found in temporal lobe epilepsy include tumours and glial hamartomas, usually quite limited in distribution to the anterior, medial, and inferior lobes (Cavanagh et al., 1958). Infarcts, the residua of inflammatory lesions, vascular abnormalities, and traumatic cicatrix are also noted. In these groups, Ammon's horn sclerosis is rarely found in association.

Hamartomas arise from a disordered cell differentiation and migration during development and resemble tumours, but are not neoplastic. They occur more frequently in the amygdala than the hippocampus and essentially represent combinations of astrocytes, oligodendrocytes, and neurones.

Finally, it should be noted that the architecture of the dendrites of hippocampal neurones has been reported abnormal in patients with temporal lobe epilepsy (Scheibel et al., 1974). Such neuronal changes are not seen in the parahippocampal gyrus (Babb et al., 1984; Scheibel, 1991).

The pathological changes are thought to relate to seizures through changes of neurotransmitter activity, especially through loss of key inhibitors such as GABA. The evidence for this in human epilepsy is circumstantial, and studies of human resected epileptic tissue have given variable results (Lloyd et al., 1985). More recently, attention has turned to abnormalities of excitatory amino acids, especially aspartate and glutamate (Meldrum, 1989). The possibility of supersensitivity of the postsynaptic receptors [either N-methyl-D-aspartate (NMDA) or non-NMDA (quisqualate or kainate) receptors] following neuronal damage is one possibility, the amino acids themselves being potentially neurotoxic.

5

Forced Normalisation and
Alternative Psychoses

In Chapter 1, the associations between epilepsy and severe psychopathology were discussed, and an emphasis was placed on two main themes. First, the increased presentation of psychopathology in epileptic patients; and second, the interictal personality changes, with the associated literature on epileptic equivalents. However, another aspect of the relationship between epilepsy and psychiatry was touched on, namely, that which suggested an antagonism.

One interpretation of this literature, albeit confused, is the idea that there could be some kind of antagonism between different illnesses. This should not be mixed up with the related idea of an antagonism of symptoms at different stages of an illness. The latter concept has a longer medical tradition. It relates to the ancient concept of "sympathy," probably first hinted at in the writings of Hippocrates and Galen (A D 131–200). Essentially, physicians struggled to explain the presence of symptoms at sites distant from an impaired body part prior to the discovery of hormones, bacteria, or even the circulation of the blood. The body was seen as an organism, and its constituent parts seen as being in sympathy (*consensus partium*). The sympathetic nerves were given a major, if not exclusive, role in this process (Riese, 1959). This doctrine of sympathy was also applied to epilepsy, and a classification into idiopathic and sympathetic epilepsy was predominant in the eighteenth century and much of the nineteenth century.

In addition to the doctrine of sympathy, there was also the concept of conversion of diseases. Ferriar (1795), who introduced the term *conversion* to medicine a century before Freud, summed it up thus: "A disease is said to be converted, when new symptoms arise in its progress, which require a different designation, and which either put a period to the original disorder, or combining with it, alter the physician's views reflecting the prognostics, or the method of cure." He went on to state: "It is so far certain, that medicines operate by producing conversions, that we perceive very considerable diseases resulting from the use of certain remedies . . . as we judge of the extinction of the original complaint, in some measure, by the increase and permanency of the remedial disease." He even anticipated convulsive therapy: "Some derangements of the mind cannot be removed, without exciting an artificial delirium" (pp. 1, 72, 73).

An earlier example, with special reference to epilepsy, comes from Willis (1667). He noted that "epilepsie is sometimes cured by the help of medicines, experience doth testifie. . . . In the meantime, as to what further belongs to the prognostication of this Disease, if it end not about the time of ripe age, neither can be driven away by the use of medicines, there happens yet a diverse event in several sick Patients, for it either ends immediately in Death, or is changed into some other Disease, to wit, the Palsie, stupiditie, or Melancholy, for the most part incurable" (p. 18).

Doubts about the specificity of epileptic psychosis occurred at the end of the nineteenth century. Marchand and Ajuriaguerra (1948) noted several authors who had reported "une sorte de substitution alternante entre le delire et la manifestation convulsive." They went on to quote a case of Parant (1895): "Cette même alternance est signalée par Parant chez une épileptique qui, sous l'influence d'un traitement bromuré, voit ses crises disparaître, mais elles sont remplacées par des troubles mentaux caractérisés par des hallucinations de l'ouïe et de la vue, des idées de persécution, de l'agitation maniaque alternant avec de la dépression; apres diminution de la dose de bromure, les acces convulsifs reparaissent et les troubles mentaux disparaissent" (p. 168).

Savage (1892) wrote: "We have met with several instances of patients who have suffered from slight attacks of epilepsy, who, having been relieved or cured of the fits of convulsions, have from that time begun to degenerate mentally, and we have elsewhere described cases in which epileptiform, if not epileptic, fits have been followed by mental improvement. . . . From some hitherto unexplained cause, severe convulsions may occur during some phases of insanity, which may be followed by recovery" (p. 455).

In the early decades of this century, the doubts about the association between epilepsy and psychosis continued, and several authors noted a low frequency of seizures in psychotics. Krapf (1928) critically reviewed the published cases, and reported six cases of his own from the Munich University Clinic. He was doubtful about the diagnosis of either the epilepsy or the schizophrenia in many instances; for example, referring to the attacks as hysteriform-tetanoid, or suggesting they were the result of hyperventilation. In his own series he either found similar objections or explained the relationship away on the grounds of latent predisposition to schizophrenia temporarily awakened.

Glaus (1931) examined over 6,000 cases from the Zurich clinic. He commented that epileptiform seizures (*epileptiformer Anfalle*) occur rarely in schizophrenia, noting references to such attacks in approximately a dozen cases, generally in catatonics in the acute stage of the illness. He thought this related to cerebral oedema. He commented that four cases had, in spite of complete absence of epileptic seizures, all the psychic features of epilepsy: "fast alle für Epilepsie bezeichnenden psychischen Eigenschaften" (p. 453). Here he was referring to hesitant speech, unctuousness, circumstantiality, perseveration, irritability, and intense affects.

However, this was a combination of schizophrenia and psychic epilepsy. This he thought of as a specific form of psychopathology rather than an organic mental illness.

Glaus was unable to support the suggestion that epilepsy and schizophrenia occurred in combination, except in the exogenous reaction form of epileptic twilight states. However, he did note that when such symptoms increase and group themselves into a characteristic pattern, then it was permissible to talk of a schizophrenic pathoplasticity, the existence of a schizophrenic constitution colouring the picture. Generally, though, he followed Bleuler, who said that in cases of epilepsy where delusions of persecution and auditory hallucinations were present, one must assume schizophrenia (Bleuler, 1911).

The arguments these authors put forward here related to the possible combination of two forms of endogenous psychoses simultaneously, obviously not compatible with ideas of a unitary psychosis. Glaus also considered the possibility of a successive combination, noting that this could occur, usually in the order of the epilepsy appearing before the psychosis. His paper (Glaus, 1931) described eight cases in which a double diagnosis was made. In four cases there was a successive combination, the schizophrenia having developed and progressed; whereas the epilepsy had not appeared for many years. Two other cases showed a similar improvement in the frequency of epileptic seizures when the schizophrenia developed. In one case he accepted the combination of epilepsy and schizophrenia. Thus, while the finding of only eight cases in 6,000 must be considered low, in seven cases, Glaus did observe either simultaneous or successive associations. The successive cases suggested some kind of antagonism, although his conclusion was that the two diseases do not significantly influence each other.

Several authors calculated the prevalence of epilepsy in schizophrenics and vice versa, the literature being reviewed by Davison and Bagley (1969). Tables 5.1 and 5.2 are taken from their review. The data on the prevalence of schizophrenia in epileptics do not reveal this to be greater than in the general population, a conclusion that Davison and Bagley found unreliable and which is discussed further in Chapter 8. Table 5.2, however, clearly shows that several other authors also noted a low prevalence rate of epilepsy in schizophrenics, but here the figures are more variable. Kraepelin (1910 through 1915), in contrast, gave the figure as 16% to 19%, although he included syncope and vertigo, thus overestimating epileptic seizures. Nonetheless, these low prevalence figures appearing in the 1920s and 1930s significantly altered the prevailing view of the relationship between schizophrenia and epilepsy from one of association to one of antagonism.

CONVULSIVE THERAPY

Laszlo von Meduna (1896–1964) first induced a seizure in a patient with severe psychiatric illness in 1934, using intramuscular camphor. He had been working in Budapest as a pupil of Professor Schaffer, and was interested in the pathology of

TABLE 5.1. *Prevalence of "Schizophrenia" in Epileptic Patients*

No. of epileptic patients	No. with schizophrenia	% ± SE	References
487	1	.2 ± .2	Ganter, 1925
2,000	15	.75 ± .2	Fürstenberg, 1949
897	7	.77 ± .3	Alström, 1950
1,806	14	.8 ± .2	Gibbs, 1952
871	6	.7 ± .4	Lorentz de Haas et al., 1956
300	2	.7 ± .5	Loeb and Giberti, 1956
1,138	6	.5 ± .2	Lorentz de Haas and Magnus, 1958
1,073	8	.75 ± .25	Bartlett, 1957

Prevalence of schizophrenia in general population 0.2% to 0.5% (Davison and Bagley, 1969).

schizophrenia. Schaffer believed that hereditary diseases were characterised by selective and specific pathological changes, and that in schizophrenia, neurones were destroyed while glial cells were unaffected. Von Meduna examined the brains of both schizophrenic and epileptic patients and noted that the changes in epilepsy were opposite to those of schizophrenia, notably with loss of few neuronal cells but with clear gliosis. He formulated a hypothesis that there was hypofunction of the glia in schizophrenia and hyperfunction in epilepsy (von Meduna, 1985). He then looked for other evidence of antagonism between the two disorders and was encouraged by Nyiro and Jablonsky (1930), who had published on the topic in 1930. Thus, in their hospital, they noted only 1.05% of epileptic patients were discharged as cured, while in epileptic patients with schizophrenia the figure was 16.5%. Von Meduna said: "From his clinical data, Professor Nyiro concluded that there was an

TABLE 5.2. *Prevalence of Epilepsy in Schizophrenic Patients*

No. of schizophrenic patients	No. with epilepsy	% ± SE	Reference
200 (females)	39	19.5 ± 2.8 ⎫	
100 (males)	14	8.0 ± 2.7 ⎬	Urstein, 1909
2,700	95	3.5 ± .35 ⎭	
347	30	8.6 ± 1.5	Giese, 1914
217	10	4.6 ± 1.4	Vorkastner, 1918
665	13	2.0 ± .5	Ballerini and Laszlo, 1964
715	20	2.7 ± .6	Yde et al., 1941
1,506	18	1.2 ± .3	Krapf, 1928
1,827	14	.77 ± .2	Peršić, 1956
537	3	.3 ± .3	Smorto and Sciorta, 1955
6,000	20	.3 ± .07	Strauss, 1929
50,000	145–165	.3 ± .02	Kat, 1937
3,242	2	.06 ± .04	de Boor, 1948
500	2	.4 ± .3	Hoch, 1943

Prevalence of epilepsy in general population 0.5%, Brewis et al., 1966 (Davison and Bagley, 1969).

antagonism between epilepsy and schizophrenia, meaning that the schizophrenic process would work against the epileptic process" (p. 54).

Nyiro followed this, injecting the blood of schizophrenics into epileptic patients, with little success. However, von Meduna concluded: "I accepted the concept of a biological antagonism between the two diseases, but I thought it worked in the opposite direction" (p. 54).

Von Meduna sought a way to create artificial convulsions and settled on camphor. Following experiments with guinea pigs, he treated his first patient in January, 1934. The results of this and other experiments are written up in a series of papers (von Meduna 1935, 1937, 1938). Although on several occasions he makes strong statements about the biological antagonism between schizophrenia and epilepsy, his precise interpretation is unclear. Thus, as noted, he relied on the results of Nyiro and Jablonsky, whose own paper (1930) noted that combinations of epilepsy and schizophrenia were by no means rare; the 16.5% figure quoted above denotes cases of a combination of the two.

Thus, it can be calculated that 95 of the series of 176 patients were considered to have only epilepsy while 81 had the combination, of whom 13 were cured. Further, von Meduna (1985) concluded: "One group of schizophrenic patients are characterised by both a tendency to self recovery and a predisposition to epileptiform attacks" (1985, p. 56).

In other words, von Meduna, while writing of antagonism, based his theory in part on cases of combinations of the two states.

In an attempt to unravel this paradox further, Wolf and Trimble (1985) noted that von Meduna was a Hungarian who wrote in German, and was not always too precise with terminology. For example, he used the terms *krankheit* (disease) and *krankheitsbild* (disorder) and *seizures* and *epilepsy* interchangeably. Further, he makes it clear that schizophrenia is an heterogenous condition with three forms: endogenous, exogenous, and exoendogenous. In the endogenous form there was no hope of any cure, but the exogenous form was that most likely to be influenced. Thus, it is suggested that he recognised the association between epilepsy and schizophrenia, but that the antagonism referred to was not that between two diseases (epilepsy and schizophrenia), but between the symptoms; namely, seizures and psychosis. This is compatible with the statements of Glaus (1931) that, in general, "in the cases of combinations of epilepsy and schizophrenia an alternating relationship is indeed the rule" (p. 499), and Wrysch (1933), who rhetorically asked: "But is it permissible to conclude from the syndromic antagonism, an antagonism of the basic disorders?"

FORCED NORMALISATION

The interest in the antagonism between psychosis and seizures was renewed at a later date from a different perspective. Heinrich Landolt, chief at the Swiss Asylum for Epileptics in Zurich, had investigated epileptic patients with paroxysmal psychiatric disorders with the newly introduced EEG. He found at least two groups of patients, one in which the EEG showed an increase in activity during the behaviour disorder, and another in which epileptic activity, present when the patient was behaviourally normal, was absent (Landolt, 1953, 1958). It is important to note his definition of psychotic episodes as "pathological mental changes which are more prolonged in time than the seizures and shorter than the chronic mental disorders seen in epilepsy" (1958, p. 91). This was limited in time, from hours to weeks, and the changes were reversible.

Landolt reported EEG investigations of 107 cases of "epileptic twilight states and psychotic episodes and 42 cases of schizophrenic attacks" (1958). He excluded catatonics and demented patients. The term *twilight states*, unlike the Anglo-Saxon meaning of an organic brain syndrome with alteration of consciousness, referred to an earlier Germanic meaning; namely, of a productive psychosis in the setting of clear consciousness, often indistinguishable from schizophrenia.

Landolt described cases of preparoxysmal dysphoria showing "regression" of the pathological EEG with what he referred to as "forced normalisation." The dysphoria indicated that "defence mechanisms against the epilepsy are set in motion" (1958, p. 101). Of the psychotic episodes, he identified four types: postparoxysmal twilight states, petit mal status, psycho-organic episodes, and productive psychotic episodes with "forced normalisation." This latter group, he suggested, formed the epileptic mania and *epilepsie larvée* of the last century. The features were polymorphous:

> They may be continuously excited, talking and even screaming uninterruptedly, restless and in constant motion, and sometimes with an excessive increase in the dynamics of ideation, with a simultaneous reduction and concentration in the range of thought. Hallucinations, illusions, delusions and compulsive acts are seen. . . . most of them feel very lucid and have the impression that their thinking is particularly clear . . . (amnesia) may be completely lacking. . . . Also within this category are the orientated and lucid twilight states in which the patients are quiet and composed, seemingly no more than slightly tense—a picture which is strikingly often almost indistinguishable from schizophrenic states (Landolt, 1958, pp. 111–112).

Landolt pointed out that these attacks could last several weeks, and may also occur in patients who have never suffered a seizure. Further, during such episodes in epileptic patients with frequent seizures, the latter were rarely expressed. The episodes could be provoked by anticonvulsant treatment and interrupted by electroconvulsive therapy (ECT), although the convulsive threshold for metrazol was elevated.

With regard to the EEG, the epileptic activity and dysrhythmias regressed during these states for their duration, the dysrhythmia returning on the recovery of mental normalcy. Landolt concluded: "Thus, these cases reveal an unmistakable correlation between the course of the psychotic process and the changes in the EEG, in that the paroxysmal focus which is active before and after the twilight state dissolves during this twilight state, and often so completely that the record is normalised. In other words, and putting it more crudely, there would seem to be epileptics who must have a pathological EEG in order to be mentally sane" (1958, p. 114).

The term *forced normalisation* has given some problems, discussed by Wolf and Trimble (1985). Originally, Landolt used the term *super-normal braking action* to express an excess of inhibition in these cases, but this was too speculative, and he preferred an empirical designation with fewer theoretical implications. He chose *forcierte Normalisierung*, but on translation to the English "forced normalisation," the meaning slightly changed. The German does not, like the English, imply some kind of definite force or mechanism. Landolt defined it thus: "Forced normalisation is the phenomenon characterised by the fact that, with the occurrence of psychotic states, the EEG becomes more normal or entirely normal as compared with previous and subsequent EEG findings" (Landolt, 1958, p. 114).

He thought it could represent the expression of a state of increased reactivity of normal tissue to the dysfunction of damaged tissue, the previous abnormality being a prerequisite for its occurrence.

Landolt also reported on the EEG of noncatatonic schizophrenics, noticing normalisation during attacks of psychosis, with temporal paroxysmal potentials or generalised or focal dysrhythmias often being noted at other times. He further supported his contentions by referring to others who had observed similar phenomena. The majority are case reports, and they are largely found in either the German or French literature of around that time. However, there were exceptions. Gibbs (1951) was experimenting with phenacemide (Phenurone) and reported intensification of psychiatric disorder in temporal lobe epilepsy on suppressing seizures. He observed that this sometimes happened with barbiturates and hydantoins, and that psychosis could be precipitated. Elimination of the drug resulted in reappearance of the seizures and resolution of the abnormal mental states. Gibbs refers to normalisation of the EEG.

Hill (1956) made similar observations but interpreted them differently. He emphasised the relevance of the onset and termination of these episodes, there being some "homoeostatic" function related to the process of recuperation and adaptation.

ALTERNATIVE PSYCHOSIS

It has to be stated that the documentation in the above literature is often poor, both with regard to the precise number of patients with differing clinical states and to the accompanying EEG profiles. However, a fair summary would be that clinically it was well-established that in some patients there was a reciprocal relationship between abnormal mental states (not necessarily always psychotic in nature) and seizures, and that, in some, there was documented EEG evidence of the forced normalisation of Landolt. Tellenbach (1965) thus introduced the term *alternative psychosis* on the grounds that it was inconvenient to always refer to "epileptic psychosis with forced normalisation of the electroencephalogram," and a shorthand term was desirable. Further, this designation did not emphasise the EEG, and was a clinical expression. Tellenbach did not imply any specific pathogeneses, but he did discuss the ideas of Landolt and put forward the suggestion that in some cases the cessation of seizures did not necessarily mean there was an arrest of the underlying disease process.

MORE RECENT STUDIES

Since the early observations of Landolt, sufficient numbers of patients with alternating psychoses have been documented to put their existence beyond doubt. Further, in some, the EEG accompaniment of forced normalisation has been recorded. One such case was reported by Stevens (1966). Glaser (1964) studied 37 patients with episodes of psychosis and temporal lobe epilepsy. He did not record true normalisation but noted, in four, intensification of psychosis along with improvement of the EEG. Using intensive EEG monitoring, including prolonged video-EEG studies, Ramani and Gumnit (1982) clearly documented forced normalisation in a 21-year-old woman with complex partial seizures who had shown a consistent inverse relationship between psychosis and seizure frequency. A similar case from the author's clinical experience is given as case 5-1:

CASE 5-1. Forced Normalisation

SJ was a 21-year-old female who had malaria at the age of 18 months and developed seizures. She had complex partial and secondarily generalised seizures that were unremitting, and were associated with an aura of fear, followed by repetitive counting to the number 16 in twos. She would then utter a scream, and lose consciousness prior to having a tonic convulsion. On coming to hospital she was having around 20 seizures a month, but occasionally had up to six seizures on a single day.

Her EEG showed slowing of the background rhythms bilaterally.

She was on carbamazepine, and was started on vigabatrin, being prescribed in increasing doses up to three grams. At that point her seizures stopped completely, but 21 days later she became lethargic and restless, and had poorly sustained attention, and tearfulness. Her behaviour became more unusual, with some disinhibition, and perseverative word play. She became preoccupied with themes of left and right, and right and wrong. She reported auditory hallucinations which made her do wrong things. She had delusions that she was born cut in half. Her sensorium was not clouded.

The EEG recorded in this psychotic state (Fig. 5-1) was considered "normalised."

The vigabatrin was slowly withdrawn, and over the next three weeks her mental state improved considerably. Following recovery, her EEG abnormalities had returned.

In her past history it was interesting that a similar experience was noted when she had become seizure-free on clobazam.

There are several more substantial investigations. In Chapter 7, the cases that have developed psychosis following temporal lobectomy are described, and in several this is associated with seizure reduction or cessation. Dongier (1959, 1960) gathered information by questionnaire from participants at a colloquium convened to examine issues on the relationship between EEG findings and psychotic states. A

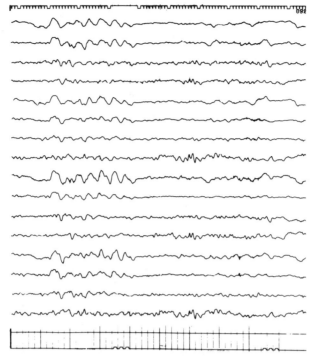

FIG. 5.1A. EEG of case 5-1 before treatment with vigabatrin.

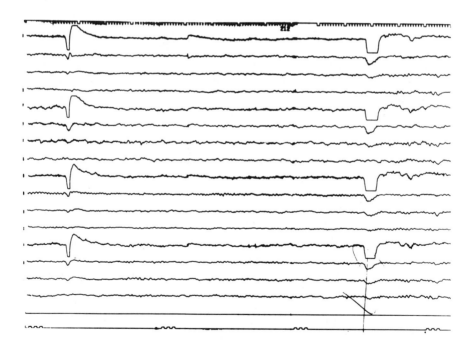

FIG. 5.1B. EEG from the same patient on vigabatrin while psychotic.

total of 536 psychotic episodes from 516 patients were documented, and 78 were identified in which there was disappearance of either a focal (50) or bisynchronous (28) discharge. Delusions were more frequent in those in which a preexisting focal discharge disappeared, and the duration of the episode was longer (several days or weeks). Paranoid behaviour was most frequent.

Palkanis et al. (1987) collected seven patients in the course of three years. They had no previous psychiatric histories, and their behavioural problems emerged shortly after starting or altering anticonvulsant therapy when seizure control was achieved. Their EEGs, abnormal before therapy change, normalised during the psychotic episodes. The patients did not have an obvious structural cause for their attacks, and neither was a long history of uncontrolled seizures a typical finding. Three were diagnosed as atypical psychosis, two as paranoid schizophrenia, and two as organic psychosis. Six had complex partial seizures, all with temporal lobe abnormalities on the EEG.

Sander et al. (1991) have recorded fifteen cases of psychosis in patients taking vigabatrin, and in five the phenomenon of alternating psychosis was observed, in some cases with EEG normalisation (see case 5-1).

These studies, and indeed the earlier work of Landolt, tended to emphasise the temporal lobe–partial seizure association with this phenomenon. However, Landolt (1963) himself wrote: "In the first years, the cortical focal epilepsies prevailed amongst those who had forced normalisation. Later, the relation turned towards the generalised epilepsies. This was clearly correlated with the progress in the treatment of petit mal. When we, in 1954, introduced the succinimide drugs there was an immediate increase in cases of forced normalisation or productive psychotic twilight states in petit mal."

This view was supported by Tellenbach (1965), and was reinforced by the reports of Fischer et al. (1965), and Roger et al. (1968). The former group described three cases with five episodes of psychosis with visual and auditory hallucinations. They had previous psychiatric histories but no prior psychotic episodes. During the ethosuximide treatment the EEG was normal. Roger et al. (1968) reviewed 20 cases from the literature, and added 15 of their own. In some, an EEG was taken in the psychotic episode, and was normalised. The development of the psychosis was seen in 4.3% of their total population, the mean age of those affected being 22 years, 8 months, the epilepsy being present for at least 14 years. Six cases had documented previous psychotic episodes. In 31 cases where information was available, there was loss of epileptic paroxysms in 22 and clinical improvement in seizures in 90% of cases. In 28 cases, EEG data were available. In 20, paroxysms totally disappeared, and in 14 the traces normalised.

Wolf (1986, 1990) has contributed several studies to this literature and has reemphasised the importance of both generalised seizures and drugs in the development of these psychoses. He investigated psychosis and related disorders in 611 patients seen in the clinic in Berlin between July, 1977 and July, 1983. There were 30 with psychotic syndromes and 7 with other episodic psychiatric disorders. Five (0.8%) showed forced normalisation. The rate was higher in generalised epilepsies (1.7%).

He also reported in his series: 19 alternative productive psychotic episodes, 12 paranoid or paranoid-hallucinatory, four catatonic-like or ecstatic, two coenaesthetic, and one delusional psychosis.

In another study of adolescents and adults with absences that required intensive treatment, he noted forced normalisation in 7.9% of cases. He emphasised that several clinical pictures may evolve, not all psychotic, as shown in Table 5.3 (Wolf and Trimble, 1985, p. 275). He noted that Tellenbach pointed out that the development of psychotic symptomatology was preceded by premonitory symptoms, especially insomnia, anxiety, feelings of oppression, and withdrawal. The insomnia, Wolf believes, is therapeutically important, since rapid administration of benzodiazepines may control this and prevent the development of the psychosis. Hysterical states (three patients developing nonepileptic "pseudoseizures") were prominent, affective disorder (two depressive, two manic), depersonalisation, and derealisation were other variants.

He noted an association between generalised idiopathic epilepsies and forced normalisation, and considered the role of anticonvulsant drugs. He accepted that most could be involved, but ethosuximide was most implicated. In his series, this was involved in all cases except one, where methsuximide was used. The phenomenon was not related to toxicity and could be seen at low doses. In contrast, sodium valproate was not involved, and cases could be switched to this without difficulty. He speculated that this may be due to the differences between the succinimides and sodium valproate on sleep, the former sometimes provoking arousal. However, this is not in accord with the report of Palkanis et al. (1987). In their series, only two patients were given succinimides and two were prescribed valproic acid.

Wolf also drew attention to social factors. He noted that unemployment was significantly higher in patients with alternative psychoses and further commented on the lack of independence in this group. The ways that social factors augmented the biological features were explained either on the grounds that social integration is a stabilising factor in a potentially psychotic patient or that better integration reflects a more stable primary personality, one better able to cope with an impending psychosis and seek help before florid manifestations develop.

TABLE 5.3. *Clinical Syndromes of Forced Normalization*

Syndrome	No. of patients
Productive psychotic episodes	19
"Prepsychotic dysphoria"	9
Hysterical episodes	5
Depressive states	3
Hypochondriacal states	3
Maniform states	2
Dysphoric states	2
Twilight state	1
Episodes of depersonalization	1

(P. Wolf, unpublished data)

PATHOGENESIS

After review of the literature, Wolf (1990) preferred the term "paradoxical normalisation" to describe the phenomenon that Landolt observed, while approving of the use of alternative psychosis. He listed 11 possible mechanisms, which were as follows:

1. The psychotic state is a reaction to the sudden cessation of seizures. This stems from suggestions that patients with epilepsy fail to adjust to the sudden loss of their illness and all of the social consequences. This fails to account for the sudden rapid onset, or the possible relationship to the succinimides. Further, the episodes are short lived, and terminated by a seizure.
2. A true "biological antagonism" exists [see below].
3. The seizure may continue, partially suppressed, with a continuing confined limbic status epilepticus, the surface EEG recordings showing only desynchronisation. It has been known for a long time that the surface records give a poor reflection of what goes on in the depths, and abnormal electrical activity in limbic structures is correlated with aggression and psychosis [see Chapter 11].
4. The generator of the epileptic discharges is still active, but the activity of the latter is propagated along unusual paths. Both this and 3 place this phenomenon into the category of an ictal status.
5. Anticonvulsants only influence seizures, and underlying metabolic processes are readjusted by them resulting in psychoses. The fact that the psychoses are sometimes terminated by a seizure gives this some support.
6. There is a reaction of the healthy parts of the brain against the epileptic focus. This is similar to Landolt's own position, and is Jacksonian.
7. Improved seizure control and the psychoses are related to activation of the Reticular Activating System.
8. Since there are reciprocal links between the Reticular Activating System (RAS) and hippocampal structures, a decrease of activity in the latter will increase RAS activity. This would not explain the state in association with control of generalised epilepsies.
9. The role of sleep [see above].
10. Increased epileptic activity is associated with increased inhibition, an electro-biological homoeostasis being renewed at a new level of tension [attributed to Christian].
11. The abnormal EEG reflects a phylogenetic immaturity of the CNS, one not adapted to contemporary environment. Archaic experiences, latently present, are activated during the normalisation [attributed to Bilz].

The problem with most of these theories is their lack of validity, or even the possibility of subjecting them to experimentation. Wolf tries to synthesise some of these, based on his own findings. He assumes that in paradoxical normalisation the epilepsy is still active but subcortical and restricted; at the same time, inhibitory processes are active. The latter lead to insomnia and possibly hypervigilance, with an associated dysphoria. At this point the psychosis is impending, but its development will depend on several other factors. These include general risk factors for psychosis, past psychotic experiences, premorbid personality, social competence, and general life situation.

BIOLOGICAL ANTAGONISM

The possible biological underpinnings of an antagonism between psychosis (especially schizophrenia-like states) and seizures have been reviewed by Reynolds (1981). He had earlier drawn attention to the fact that patients with epilepsy receiving anticonvulsant drugs became folate deficient, and that this was greater in those with severe psychiatric illness or dementia. Further, folate is convulsant, emphasising how folate-deficient states could lead to a diminution of seizures in the presence of a psychosis.

Reynolds gives other examples of antagonisms, shown in Table 5.4 (Reynolds 1981, p. 275). These include methionine and methionine-sulfoximine. Trimble (1977) suggested that dopamine may be involved. Thus, antipsychotic drugs are dopamine antagonists, and are known to provoke seizures (see p. 150). Dopamine agonists both increase the intensity of psychotic symptoms or can precipitate a psychosis while also possessing some anticonvulsant properties (Fig. 5.2). However, alternative hypotheses might be constructed using GABA or perhaps a peptide.

In general, the neurotransmitter-based hypotheses have more merit for the kind of events that Landolt described, in the sense that changes in folate metabolism are not rapid and short lived, while a switch in neurochemical status within specified neurotransmitter pathways can occur rapidly and are seen, for example, following the administration of a multitude of psychotropic drugs.

CONCLUSIONS

The literature reviewed in this chapter establishes one clear link between epilepsy and psychosis, namely, that revealed through the phenomenon of forced normalisation. It also clarifies a misunderstanding of the associations between the two;

TABLE 5.4. *Evidence of Biological Antagonism Between Epilepsy and Schizophrenia*

Agent	Epilepsy	Schizophrenia
Anticonvulsant drugs, barbiturates	Therapeutic	?Aggravation
Phenothiazines	Convulsant	Therapeutic
Methionine	?Therapeutic	Aggravation
Methionine-sulfoximine	Convulsant	?Therapeutic
EEG	'Forced normalisation' (Landolt)	'Homeostatic' (Hill)
Folic acid	?Aggravation	??

? implies need for more substantial evidence (Reynolds, 1968).

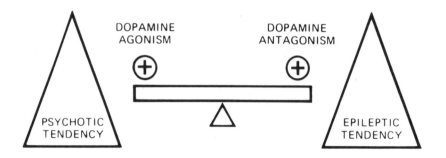

AGONISTS eg. L.DOPA, PIRIBEDIL, APOMORPHINE, NOMIFENSINE

ANTAGONISTS eg. PHENOTHIAZINES, HALOPERIDOL, PIMOZIDE

FIG. 5.2. Relationship between epilepsy, psychosis, and dopamine.

namely, that the antagonism is between symptoms viewed longitudinally rather than between two independent disease entities. Indeed, neither epilepsy nor schizophrenia can be viewed as diseases, they are both syndromes with several underlying disease processes, some of which seem common to both.

It is often denied that forced normalisation (and its clinical counterpart, alternative psychosis), occurs, probably with good reason. Thus, it is certainly rarer than made out by Landolt, and studies are few and far between. It is difficult to document such cases precisely, and EEG recordings often cannot be obtained. However, another less enlightened reason to ignore such findings is that their presence reveals too closely the association between seizures and psychosis, and has a profound effect on treatment. Thus, if in some patients suppression of seizures provokes psychopathology, it means that seizures and epilepsy are not synonymous, and that an understanding of the epileptic process and its treatment goes far beyond control of seizures. Tellenbach referred to the writings of Landolt (1963) when he suggested: "Today, however, it seems to us more and more that the treatment of epilepsy on the whole has its limits insofar as the efficiency or impetuosity of the anticonvulsant action of some new drugs places us in certain cases more and more before the alternative: mental illness or epilepsy, seizures or madness. And, of course, it is still better to have seizures than to be mentally ill."

6

Auras, Ictal Events, and Peri-Ictal Psychoses

When considering the relationship between epilepsy and psychiatry, mental changes associated with the ictus are of considerable importance. On the theoretical level, ictally related psychoses provide clear evidence for direct neurophysiological links between psychotic states and altered brain states. There are few active clinicians who have not encountered such clinical pictures, yet many still are unable to accept that there are psychiatric consequences of epilepsy, especially psychoses. Brief consideration of the auras of partial seizures and the clinical presentations of complex partial seizure status must make these doubts untenable. At the practical level, ictal mental changes may be mistaken for an alternative psychiatric diagnosis, notably schizophrenia, and lead to inappropriate management.

In this chapter, three aspects of ictally related psychotic episodes will be considered. First, the auras, notably of simple and complex partial seizures; second, status epilepticus; and third, postictal psychoses.

AURAS

The term *aura* seems to have derived originally from the Greek for "a breeze," and to have early been recognised as indicating the beginning of the seizure. Initially the aura was viewed as a sensory phenomenon, but by the nineteenth century it had broadened to include motor and psychical phenomena. Griesinger (1857) noted that there were many epileptic conditions in which "psychical disorder" could be recognised during the attack. It was Hughlings Jackson, however, who so clearly delineated the cognitive and emotional aspects of the aura with his descriptions, notably of the affliction of Dr. Z.

Hughlings Jackson (1880, 1881) referred to the "intellectual aura," which he thought to be a poor term, and described it thus: "The state is often like that occasionally experienced by healthy people as a feeling of 'reminiscence.' . . . It is sometimes called 'dreamy feelings,' or is described as 'dreams mixing up with present thoughts,' 'double consciousness,' 'feeling of being somewhere else,' 'as if I went back to all that occurred in my childhood.' Sometimes there is a definite elaborate vision . . . these are all voluminous mental states and yet of different kinds" (p. 199).

Hughlings Jackson identified these states as usually being associated with "sensations of smell, and epigastric sensations, and with the supposed gustatory movements" and speculated on their origin:

> They cannot be owing to an epileptic discharge. It would be a remarkably well-directed and distributed epileptic discharge which would give rise to the exceedingly compound mental state of being somewhere else. Besides, it must not be forgotten that there very often is along with the dreamy state one of the crude subjective sensations mentioned. It is scarcely likely that one thing, an epileptic discharge, should be the physical condition for a sudden stench in the nose—a crude sensation—and also the physical condition for an infinitely more elaborate psychical state. I submit that the former occurs during the epileptic discharge, and that the latter is owing to but slightly raised activity of healthy nervous arrangements consequent on 'loss of control'—possibly of some in the cerebral hemisphere opposite the one, which I believe to be nearly always the right, in which the discharge begins (1880/81 p. 200).

Hughlings Jackson went on to identify the anatomical localisation for the crude sensations as the uncinate region of the temporal lobe, suggesting they could be referred to as the "Uncinate Group of Fits."

Thus, in his analysis of patients with such auras, which included in some of his cases both illusions and hallucinations, Jackson not only outlined the existence of a form of epilepsy later recognised as temporal lobe epilepsy, but he also noted the association with "psychical" changes, the anatomical derivation, and speculated on the mechanism of the development of the mental symptoms.

Literature has provided us with some examples of such seizures with psychotic contents. The case of such mystics as Saint Paul of Tarsus has been mentioned (p. 3), as has that of Dostoievski (pp. 9–10). The correspondence of Flaubert contains the following reference to an acute ictal experience: "I who have heard through closed doors people talking in low tones thirty paces away (hallucinations of sound), across whose abdomen one may see the viscera throbbing, and who have sometimes felt in the space of a minute a million thoughts, images, and combinations of all kinds throwing themselves into my brain at once, as it were a lighted squib of fireworks" (Spratling, 1904, p. 466).

The first major study of auras was that of Gowers (1901). The second edition of his textbook *Epilepsy and Other Chronic Convulsive Diseases* is based on over 2,000 cases, of which some aura existed in 57%. Psychical auras were recorded in 4.6%, although he was not able to confirm an association to the epigastric aura suggested by Hughlings Jackson. He noted associations with taste or olfactory auras. He also reported complex visual and auditory hallucinations which he classified separately from psychical auras.

Lennox and Cobb (1933) reported on a large sample of 750 patients, the proportion reporting auras (56%) being similar to that reported by Gowers. Subjective, psychic auras accounted for 12.1%, visual for 6.8% and auditory for 1.7%. Lennox said of some of the psychic auras that, in them, patients "may seem to balance on the edge of another world" (Lennox and Lennox, 1960, vol. 1, p. 179).

Penfield and Jasper (1954) divided psychical seizures into four groups: 1) illusions, 2) emotions, 3) hallucinations, and 4) forced thinking. The first group includes visual (e.g., micropsia and macropsia) and auditory phenomena, déjà vu and related events, and illusions of emotion, most often fear. The hallucinations are visual and auditory, the latter consisting sometimes of a single voice, sometimes many, and often speaking to the patient. In general, they reported that emotional seizures emanate from discharges deep in the sylvian fissure or on the undersurface of the temporal lobe, while hallucinations are temporal or temporoparietal in origin. In their extensive summary of such ictal experiences, Penfield and Perot (1963) give the laterality as in Table 6.1.

Williams (1956) attempted further localisation of such seizure experiences in a study of 100 patients with epilepsy who experienced emotion as part of their seizure. Anterior and middle temporal sites were particularly common, although this localisation was far greater (100%) for those with an aura of fear. Depression was rather poorly localised, being diffuse or nonlocalised in 52%. In this series, feelings of pleasure, including elation, occurred in nine patients. Paranoid feelings were also noted, similar auras having been reported by others (MacLean, 1990).

Bingley (1958) examined the ictal mental experiences of 90 patients with temporal lobe epilepsy. "Dreamy states" were recorded in 32% of cases, and were more common with a lesion in the nondominant lobe (58% as compared with 24% in the dominant hemisphere). Auditory illusions and hallucinations were noted in 18% and visual phenomena in 18%. Anxiety was the most common ictal experience, being reported by 36% of cases, often being associated with epigastric sensations. Three patients had ictal depression, and four had euphoric states.

More recent studies of auras include those of Gupta et al. (1983), and of Taylor and Lochery (1987). The former examined 290 patients with complex partial seizures and EEG evidence of site of seizure focus. Auras were reported in 64% of the total, and psychic and autonomic auras were more common with right-sided abnormalities. Taylor and Lochery (1987) analysed the auras of 88 patients with temporal lobe epilepsy who had received temporal lobectomy. They divided the auras into three types, namely, simple primitive, special senses, and intellectual. Fear was

TABLE 6.1. *Laterality of Ictal Hallucinations*

	Nondominant	Dominant	Total
Auditory	4	8	12
Visual	15	6	21
Combined	3	8	11
Unclassified	2	7	9
Total	24	29	53

(Penfield and Perot, 1963, p. 676)

noted twice as commonly with mesial temporal sclerosis, intellectual auras occurring exclusively in males with a verbal IQ above 100. There was no relationship between the content of the auras and the presence of psychosis. This was in contrast to the study of Hermann et al. (1982a) in which patients with an aura of ictal fear scored higher in interictal psychopathology than others. This is considered further on page 114.

Kanemoto and Janz (1989) considered the temporal sequence of auras in 143 patients with complex focal seizures. Epigastric auras and illusions of familiarity were the most frequent, followed by ictal aphasia, anxiety, and thought disorder. Left-sided foci predominated for aphasia and thought disorder; nonspecific auras, anxiety, and epigastric sensations were almost exclusively found at the start of the aura sequence; thought disorder was intermediate; aphasia was always at the end.

STIMULATION STUDIES

To complement the clinical data obtained from an analysis of aura experiences, several groups have carried out brain stimulation with implanted cerebral electrodes, largely in epileptic patients, in an endeavour to explore localisation further. A pioneer was Heath (1975), whose extensive studies highlighted an area in the rostral medial forebrain (referred to by his group as the septal region) as a key area for emotional expression. This encompasses several structures including the septal nuclei, the olfactory tubercle, the subcallosal gyrus, the rostrum of the corpus callosum, the subcallosal fasciculus, and the piriform cortex. This forms part of a system, including sites along the MFB, that on stimulation lead to pleasurable feelings. Adversive emotions were recorded with stimulation of the hippocampus and amygdala, periaqueductal sites in the mesencephalon and in the medial hypothalamus.

Penfield also carried out stimulation studies although, unlike Heath, he did not employ extensive depth studies (Penfield and Perot, 1963). He referred to hallucinations of things previously seen or heard with stimulation as experiential responses. These phenomena could be simple or complex, were usually either visual or auditory, and were recognised by the patient as coming from the past. Illusions were also evoked, for example, déjà vu and automatisms. Of the latter, Penfield noted that the site of production was beneath the uncus, and the stimulus had to be strong enough to provoke an afterdischarge. Experiential phenomena derived exclusively from discharge in the temporal cortex.

Visual illusions and illusions of familiarity were predominantly associated with stimulation of the nondominant temporal lobe, auditory illusions being evoked bilaterally, chiefly from the first temporal convolutions. Penfield identified the primary auditory sensory area as the anterior one of the transverse gyri of Heschl within the sylvian fissure, just posterior to the insula. Most importantly, he stated: "The points from which stimulation produced experiences which were chiefly auditory have a clear tendency to appear in the neighbourhood of the auditory sensory cortex but never in it" (1963, p. 685).

With regard to experiential responses, Penfield reported they occurred in only 7.7% of patients, while ictal spontaneous experiential hallucinations were reported in 10%. Auditory experiential phenomena were the most frequently encountered and derived from a limited area on the lateral and superior surface of the first temporal convolutions. Visual phenomena were elicited from a similar area, although the zone implicated extended more posteriorly on the nondominant side, covering the area devoted to speech on the dominant side. The laterality of these responses is given in Table 6.2.

In these stimulation studies, in contrast to the spontaneous ictal experiences, there is an excess of nondominant responses. Whether this reflected the fact that more patients had nondominant operations (15 left, 25 right) or relates to some fundamental difference between ictal and stimulated experiences is unclear.

Halgren and colleagues (1978) pointed out how few patients actually reported experiential phenomena, and how stimulation at the same point at different times may evoke different responses. The role of the patient's personality in the subsequent evoked experience had been commented on by several authors (Rayport and Ferguson, 1974), the hallucinations being symbolically related to ongoing psychodynamic processes. Such factors were ignored in Penfield's studies, as indeed were attempts to confirm the veracity of many of the patients' evoked "memories."

Halgren et al. (1978) noted that mental phenomena were rarely evoked until the strength of the stimulus was sufficient to induce widespread evoked responses and afterdischarges, and then the type of experience was related to patient-specific variables such as personality rather than the precise position of the stimulating electrode. They stereotactically implanted electrodes bilaterally into the amygdala, hippocampus, and the hippocampal gyrus in 36 patients who were candidates for surgery for epilepsy. Stimulation of posterior electrodes elicited mental phenomena only one quarter as often as did stimulation of anterior electrodes, but no laterality effect was noted. The category of mental phenomenon recorded was related to the particular patient stimulated rather than the electrode site. They tested specific hypotheses relating to personality by using the Minnesota Multiphasic Personality Inventory (MMPI). Patients who experienced fear or anxiety scored higher on the Pt

TABLE 6.2. *Laterality of Experiential Responses*

	Nondominant	Dominant	Total
Auditory	42	24	66
Visual	28	10	38
Combined	13	9	22
Unclassified	8	4	12
Total	91	47	138

(Penfield and Perot, 1963, p. 670)

(psychasthenia) scale, while those with memory-like or dreamlike hallucinations scored higher on the Sc (schizophrenia) scale.

Gloor and colleagues (1982) have also reported on the elicitation of experiential phenomena with brain stimulation. They repeated some of Penfield's observations, but clearly located the origin of the experiential phenomena in limbic structures. Thirty-five patients with intracerebral depth electrodes were stimulated, and in the majority it was noted that their seizures originated in one or the other temporal lobe. In contrast to Penfield's data, 52% of their subjects had a positive response, fear being the most common. The location of the seizures or afterdischarges associated with experiential phenomena is shown in Table 6.3. In 37 instances discharges were confined to limbic structures, in only two was the temporal neocortex alone involved, and then it was not lateral but in the depth. In other words, the phenomena were associated with seizures or afterdischarges that involved either the limbic system alone or limbic and neocortical structures. Even complex visual hallucinations were reported with limbic stimulation alone. They also noted an anteroposterior gradient, the amygdala being the most favoured site, but emphasised that afterdischarges were not crucial.

The mechanism of the development of experiential phenomena has been discussed by several authors. Hughlings Jackson (1879) referred to "removal of higher centres" in relationship to the aura. Penfield and Perot (1963) took a clear localisationist view that the site of the electrode was crucial, and gave prime importance to cortical grey matter. For them, interpretive cortex had activating connections with part of the record of the stream of consciousness in which hearing and vision were prominent, the latter lying at a distance from the temporal cortex itself. Halgren and colleagues suggested that either stimulation excited neural elements afferent and efferent to the temporal lobe, or the temporal lobe may be put temporarily out of action, leading to deficits but also to other mental phenomena as interactions with other ongoing cerebral events occur. Disruption of the function of the medial temporal lobe alters the ongoing activity of the rest of the brain, which then leads to consideration of spontaneous neural patterns present at the time of stimulation, in-

TABLE 6.3. *Location of Seizures or Afterdischarges Associated with Experiential Phenomena*

Location	No. of observations
Amygdala	5
Hippocampus	5
Parahippocampal gyrus	1
Temporal neocortex	2
Amygdala + hippocampus	15
Amygdala + hippocampus + parahippocampal gyrus	11
Amygdala + hippocampus + parahippocampal gyrus + temporal neocortex	>49

(Glorr et al., 1982, p. 137)

fluenced by the patient's ongoing concerns. Complex hallucinations are explained as an example of the latter mechanism. They suggest, on the basis of known anatomy and animal investigations, that the hippocampus or its disruption is crucial for the hallucinatory experience.

Gloor (1991) argues against the necessity to invoke cortical change, emphasising the primacy of the limbic system. The latter gives "experiential immediacy to neo-cortically elaborated percepts, attaching motivational and emotional significance" (p. 20). The latter, he conjectures, may be a precondition for the percept to be consciously experienced. He suggests that the experiential phenomena are a positive expression of the functions of the temporal lobes, not interference or paralysis of such functions. Thus, they are aura, and occur only at the beginning of the seizure; if they were related to paralysis they would to be present postictally as well. Further, since the temporal lobes are the anatomical substrata of such phenomena, it is illogical to consider their appearance as secondary to inactivation.

In conclusion, the data on auras and stimulation show that patients with epilepsy have experiences that form part of traditional psychopathology, especially hallucinations. Insight is usually maintained, and specific Schneiderian phenomena have not been recorded, but in all probability have not been examined for. Schizophreniform experiences such as forced thinking and thought disorder are noted. Karagulla and Robertson (1955) many years ago noted the similarity between the ictal experiences of epileptic patients and the symptoms of schizophrenia.

Laterality effects have only been consistently reported for "dreamy states" including déjà vu phenomena (although not by Kanemota and Janz, 1989), and there is some discrepancy between findings on stimulation and spontaneous ictal phenomena in the same patient. This may relate to the observation that there is a lower frequency of evoked phenomena from diseased as opposed to nondiseased lobes, the natural seizure being a better stimulus in the former. Several authors have argued that the limbic system, especially the hippocampus and the amygdala, are crucial for the development of experiential phenomena, but the variability between patients (or with the same patient at different times) argues against a strict localisationist interpretation of the events.

STATUS EPILEPTICUS

The term *status epilepticus* is generally reserved for serial seizures in which the patient does not gain consciousness between attacks. Although the paradigm is that of generalised tonic-clonic attacks, it is now recognised that partial seizures and absence attacks can present as status. Curiously, status epilepticus was not recognised until the early nineteenth century and was not a notable cause of death in epilepsy until the end of that century (Hunter, 1959, 1960). The term *nonconvulsive status* is now used to refer to absence status and complex partial status of frontal or temporal origin.

Absence Status

Lennox appears to have introduced the term *petit mal status* (Lennox and Lennox, 1960), and of 1,039 cases of petit mal reported by Gibbs and Gibbs (1952), 2.6% had a history of status. It is characterised by a spectrum from subtle alterations of consciousness to more obvious torpor or stupor, and there is often accompanying periorbital movements with rapid eye blinking in phases and observable myoclonic jerks. Patients are disoriented, may perseverate, and appear apathetic. Status usually occurs in patients with a known history of generalised seizures, and while most episodes are seen under the age of 20, sudden onset in later life is reported (Schwartz and Scott, 1971), in some cases with no prior history of seizures (Ellis and Lee, 1973).

The EEG reveals generalised discharges of a typical 3 cps spike-wave variety. These episodes may be frequent and last a variable time from minutes to several weeks. After a number of years, there may be an associated behavioural disturbance during the episodes, especially with accompanying deterioration of the EEG. If the condition remains unrecognised, then the latter may be misattributed and inappropriate treatments initiated.

Lugaresi et al. (1971) draw the distinction between this relatively pure form and those patients with atypical spike-wave discharges. In the latter, the episodes may be associated with severe psychiatric disturbances with associated hallucinations and delusions. Ellis and Lee (1978) described several cases with delusions, hallucinations, and thought disorder in the setting of an encephalopathy, emphasising in some cases the continuum with postictal states or, rather, the difficulty of making such clear distinctions in some patients when EEG and other criteria are taken into account. Wells (1975) reported a case of a patient with psychotic depression and an EEG showing frequent bursts of 2 cps spike-wave activity.

Complex Partial Seizure Status

Partial status may present in a variety of forms, but that associated with psychotic behaviour is inevitably complex partial, and the focus arises from either the temporal or the frontal lobes. Interestingly, case reports are rare. The onset is sudden but may occur following a bout of generalised seizures, sometimes with a lucid interval before the onset of the psychosis. In the latter cases the EEG is likely to show a more generalised change. Patients have varying degrees of confusion which, in some cases, is detected only with careful testing. In the various reports in which EEG documentation is available, the confusional state is most marked upon (e.g., Engel et al., 1978). Automatisms, fugues, and intense panic or fear are reported, as are hallucinations, delusions, and illusions. States resembling schizophrenia, with typical thought disturbances and Schneiderian first rank symptoms, can occur. An example of the author's is given in case 6.1:

CASE 6.1

A 22-year-old man, with a history of complex partial and generalized tonic-clonic seizures since the age of 3 1/2, had the sudden onset of "indescribable feelings" that rays were being passed through his body in order to sterilize him. Subsequently he heard voices criticizing him in both the second and third persons and was admitted to a psychiatric hospital with an acute psychosis, diagnosed as schizophrenia.

While under observation, his mental state was variable, at times being torpid and hardly responsive, at other times restless and demanding to go home. As he became communicative, it was clear he had a florid paranoid psychosis with schizophreniform features. An EEG was carried out, showing frequent sharp waves on the right side with phase reversals at the right sphenoidal electrode which were almost continuous (Fig. 6.1).

The patient's mental state responded promptly to intravenous diazepam, as did the electroencephalographic disturbance. Over the ensuing months he was readmitted to a mental hospital on several occasions with acute onset episodes of a similar psychosis.

Wieser and colleagues (1985) provided a comprehensive report on four patients examined with depth electrodes. They had variable behavioural patterns, two with personality changes such as stickiness, aggressiveness, and personal neglect; others having hallucinations, illusions, and dream-like feelings. Recurrent to continuous seizure discharges were recorded from either limbic or limbic and neocortical structures. Importantly, in two of their cases, including one with a personality change similar to that described by Geschwind (see p. 119), no impairment of consciousness was noted, although using sophisticated tachistoscopic methods, a circumscribed alteration of cognitive performance was shown, corresponding to an inefficiency on the side of the limbic focus.

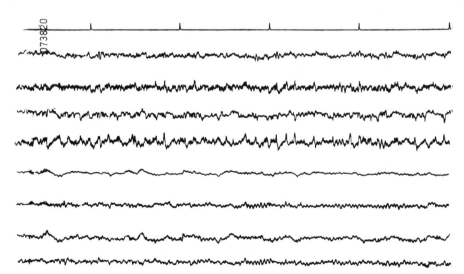

FIG. 6.1. Showing the EEG of case 6.1. The top four leads are from the right, and three and four represent sphenoidal recordings. The patient demonstrated very frequent sharp waves with phase reversals at the right sphenoidal electrodes.

Hurwitz et al. (1985) provided evidence of EEG-behavioural correlation in a 33-year-old right-handed woman with independent left- and right-sided temporal lobe discharges. Using continuous EEG recordings, it was reported that after left-sided discharges she became dysphasic and depressed and had auditory hallucinations of a schizophrenic nature. With right-sided episodes she became disinhibited and hypomanic.

Gillig et al. (1988) provided similar information in a case report of a 32-year-old man with ictal mania. Associated with the onset of rhythmic slowing in the right parietal and right posterior temporal regions, he became agitated, sang and spoke unintelligible phrases, and experienced auditory and visual hallucinations. Pressure of speech, clanging, and neologisms were also reported.

POSTICTAL PSYCHOSES

In many cases the distinction between the ictus itself and the postictal phase is hard to distinguish. While it is clear that the aura is the start of the ictus, the various behavioural manifestations reported thereafter are perhaps best referred to as peri-ictal, thus emphasising a relationship to the electrophysiological events of the ictus. Likewise, distinguishing the ictal from the interictal phases can sometimes be an equally fruitless exercise.

Although, generally, "ictal" refers to short-lived events, some of the peri-ictal behavioural manifestations can last hours or even days. The evidence that they should be considered ictally related is the onset coincident with the ictus and persisting electrophysiological disturbances as reflected on the EEG.

In clinical practice, postictal psychoses are the most commonly observed epileptic psychotic events. They emerge from the ictas with confusion, automatisms, wandering, and often inappropriate behaviour. A comprehensive study of 52 cases was reported by Levin (1952). They tended to be older than his cases without "clouded states," the peak age of distribution being 30 to 40 years. Hallucinations (mainly auditory) were reported in 36% and delusions (mainly persecutory) in 24%. Where data were available, had their abnormal mental states developed within 24 hours of a seizure in 17 of 23 cases but in 4 it was 1 to 2 days, and in 2 it was 2 to 7 days. In most (14 out of 21), 2 or more seizures heralded the disorder.

More recently, Logsdail and Toone (1988) have provided a more detailed phenomenological account of postictal psychoses. They retrospectively examined the records of 14 cases that fulfilled these criteria:

a: An episode of confusion or psychosis manifested immediately upon a seizure, or emerged within a week of the return of apparently normal mental function.

b: A minimum length of 24 hours, and a maximum of 3 months.

c: The mental state was characterised by one of the following:

    1: clouding of consciousness, disorientation or delirium.

    2: delusions, hallucinations in clear consciousness.

    3: a mixture of 1 and 2.

d: No evidence of the following extraneous factors which might have contributed to the abnormal mental state:

1: anticonvulsant toxicity.

2: a previous history of interictal psychosis.

3: EEG evidence of minor status.

4: recent history of head injury, or alcohol or drug intoxication.

The phenomenology of the mental state was rated using the Syndrome Check List (SCL) derived from the Present State Examination (PSE) of Wing and colleagues (1974). Five patients had one psychotic episode, six had two to four, and three had multiple attacks. The mean age of onset of epilepsy was 16.7 years, and onset of the psychosis was 32.2 years. Three patients had primary generalised epilepsy causing generalised tonic-clonic seizures, the rest had complex partial seizures with intermittent secondary generalisation. Seizure control was variable, but in 86% of cases there was a clear history of an increase in generalised seizure frequency prior to the onset of the psychosis, usually in a cluster. In 78% there was a lucid interval lasting from 1 to 6 days (mean 2.5) in which the mental state was normal after recovery from the major seizures.

The phenomenology of the psychoses was pleomorphic, some patients displaying obvious confusion. Mood was markedly abnormal in 75%, being elevated, depressed, or both. Fifty percent had paranoid delusions, while auditory and visual hallucinations were both common.

With regard to PSE categorisation, the final results revealed four with schizophrenic psychosis, three manic and mixed affective psychoses, and four paranoid psychoses. Three were rated under other psychoses. Six patients were judged to be seriously behaviourally disturbed, including one suicide attempt and two who were physically aggressive.

Follow-up data were available on all patients ranging from 3 months to 8 years. Four had died, and three had developed or were developing a chronic interictal psychosis.

In discussing their cases, the authors make the point that "mental state phenomena occur that are identical to those which are found in, and are diagnostic of, the functional psychoses, and they occur frequently in clear consciousness" (p. 251).

They note that these postictal states have several features in common with interictal psychoses (see Chapter 8): namely, lack of family history for psychosis, overrepresentation of complex partial seizures, and the similar interval between the age of onset of the epilepsy and the age of onset of the psychosis.

The observations of Toone et al. on the relative frequency of affective changes receive support from the subsequent reporting of five cases of hypomania following seizures derived from the temporal lobes (Barczak, et al. 1988; Byrne, 1988). In two, religiosity was a prominent part of the mental state. Interestingly, all were male, had had a flurry of seizures, and had a right-sided focus of origin of their seizures.

Savard et al. (1987) reported nine cases of postictal psychosis after complex partial seizures which followed an increase in seizure activity in seven. Two of their series had only unilateral seizures; the rest were bilateral. In seven the psychosis was paranoid, while in two it was schizophreniform. They speculated that the phenomenon was analogous to motor, memory, and sensory abnormalities that occur following seizures; namely, a variant of Todd's phenomenon.

CONCLUSIONS

From the data reviewed in this chapter it is clear that the acute electrophysiological disturbance of the ictus is associated with mental state changes which represent psychopathological phenomena. Further, in some patients a bout of status epilepticus (especially complex partial seizure status) can lead to a clinical state in which consciousness is minimally clouded, and clinical pictures resembling major psychiatric disorders such as schizophrenia are seen. Finally, postictal psychoses are not uncommon, again presenting with recognised psychopathological pictures which sometimes merge out of the ictal states but often seem to arise following a flurry of seizures and a subsequent lucid interval. The changes of affect, especially associated with hypomanic presentations, in association with right-sided epileptic activity, are striking. Some patients go on to develop chronic interictal psychoses, a theme taken up further in Chapter 8.

7

Postoperative Psychoses

There are several operative procedures now carried out on patients with epilepsy, although such interventions are restricted to those with severe intractable seizures. In the main, focal resections, corpus callostomy, and major resections are the preferred procedures, although selected lesions in stereotactic targets, especially into limbic and subcortical sites, have also been carried out. Cerebellar stimulation is also on occasions performed. The literature on psychosis relates almost exclusively to temporal lobectomies, and this literature is reviewed in this chapter.

HISTORY OF SURGERY

With the exception of earlier trephining and decompression techniques, the first modern neurosurgical operation on a patient with epilepsy was carried out by Rickman Goodlee in 1884, and the acclaimed work of Victor Horsley (1886) was soon to follow.

Burckhardt (1891) did temporal lobe resections on two psychotic patients without epilepsy in attempt to alleviate hallucinations. In this century, Forester and later Penfield laid the foundations of modern-day temporal lobectomy operations. Initially only a minority of epileptic patients had this operation, the main resections being carried out on potentially identifiable cortical scars or tumours, often extratemporal in origin. In 1955, Penfield and Paine reported that of 68 patients with temporal lobe seizures operated on between 1939 and 1949, only three had no visible abnormality. Gibbs apparently persuaded Percival Bailey to operate on patients with temporal lobe epilepsy on the basis of EEG findings, the first operation under the guidance of electrocorticography being performed in March, 1947. Focal removal of an identified spiking focus led to excision operations of the discharging temporal lobe.

OPERATIVE TECHNIQUES

Many earlier surgeons followed the techniques developed by Penfield at the Montreal Neurological Institute, in which the anterior part of the temporal lobe was removed using suction (Penfield and Jasper, 1954), rarely beyond Labbé's vein (the posterior anastomotic vein which connects the middle cerebral vein with tributaries of the transverse sinuses). Murray Falconer at the Guy's-Maudsley Neurosurgical Unit removed the temporal lobe anterior to Labbé's vein in one piece. This involved approximately 6 to 8 cm of tissue which included the uncus, parts of the amygdala, and the anterior 2 to 3 cm of the hippocampus. The superior temporal gyrus was usually spared, especially on the dominant side, excisions being less extensive in that hemisphere. A major advantage was the preservation of the temporal lobe for pathological studies (Fig. 7.1).

This method became modified as new technology permitted more elaborate pre- and intraoperative workup. The latter included the use of stereotactically implanted depth or subdural electrodes, and advanced neuroradiology with computerised tomography (CT), magnetic resonance imaging (MRI), SPECT, or positron emission tomography (PET). Neuropsychological techniques such as Wada testing, precise memory testing, and the location of cortical language areas by intraoperative mapping have all helped to minimise postoperative psychological impairments.

Selective removal of the hippocampus and amygdala has also been carried out (Niemeyer, 1958; Wieser, 1988). Following his classification of complex partial seizures into five types, Wieser found that 70% were mediobasal. He surmised that the hippocampus and amygdala, as important relays in the limbic system, were crucial to the genesis of the seizure. Using microsurgical techniques, Yasargil developed his selective operation in which the amygdala, hippocampus, and parahippocampal gyrus are selectively removed.

RESULTS OF SURGERY

Seizures

There are several reviews of the results of temporal lobectomy and its variants (Jensen, 1975; Engel, 1987). The results vary, dependent on the centre reporting the data and on the length of follow-up. Generally, the longer the follow-up, the more patients will fall into a category of having recurrent seizures. Engel reviewed the outcome of temporal lobectomy in 2,336 patients from 40 centres worldwide, and reported that 55% were seizure-free, follow-up ranging from 2 to 37 years. However, there was a considerable variability, from 26% to 80%, and the variance of those not improved ranged from 6% to 29%. Polkey (1988) gave figures for 90 Maudsley patients of 25% seizure-free, while Rasmussen (1983) quotes a figure of 37% for 894 evaluable patients with nontumoural lesions and 46% for 176 tumoural resections in the Montreal series. The UCLA results given by Crandall (1987) are based on an evaluation of best outcome being those seizure-free or having rare seizures; 51% of 59 patients were in this category for a pre–1977 series, compared with 92% of 12 cases after 1979. If occasional seizures are accepted as a good result, then the equivalent figure for the Maudsley series is 58% and for Montreal are 50% and 46% for nontumoural and tumoural cases, respectively.

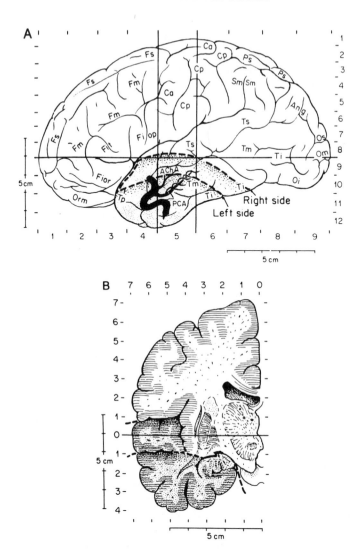

FIG. 7.1. Falconer en bloc anterior temporal lobectomy. **A:** Arteries at risk are the anterior choroidal artery and the posterior cerebral artery and its branches. The resection of lesser extent refers to the nondominant lobe. **B:** Coronal view of resection. (From Engel, 1987, with permission.)

A long-term follow-up study of the Falconer series has been reported by Bruton (1988). Of 234 cases, 32% were free of seizures for at least 5 years; a further 36% had their attacks substantially reduced.

For selective amygdalohippocampectomy, Wieser (1988) reported that 62% of 181 patients were seizure-free.

In general, outcome is better for patients with radiological evidence of non-atrophic temporal lobe pathology or in those with a history of a complicated convulsion in early childhood and evidence of a unilateral discharging focus, and with an

IQ over 90 (Oxbury and Adams, 1989). Bruton (1988) examined outcome in relation to pathological findings in detail and reported the best improvement in those with alien tissue lesions (a combination of glial lesions, neuronoglial lesions, and vascular abnormalities) and Ammon's horn sclerosis, especially those with mixed glial lesions and the ganglioglial type of neuronoglial lesion. Calcification within alien tissue lesions was also a good prognostic. In those with no apparent pathology, the results of surgery were poor.

Psychological Tests

It is accepted that psychological testing is an integral part of the preoperative workup for surgery. It was early recognised that the structures involved in temporal lobe discharges, especially the hippocampus, were important parts of a complex system subserving memory, and that the catastrophic consequences of bilateral destruction of medial temporal structures resulting in an amnestic syndrome were apparent in a few early cases (Terzian, 1958). One reason for evaluation is, therefore, to specifically test memory function and its relationship to any identified lesion site. A further important use of neurophysiological testing is to aid with identification of the side of the brain which is involved in seizure generation; this can be correlated with other data to accurately localise lesion sites.

The consequences of temporal lobectomy for neuropsychological (especially memory) function have been reviewed by several authors (Milner, 1966; Dodrill, 1988). In 1957, Milner and colleagues described a severe anterograde and retrograde amnesia in an epileptic patient, H.M., following bilateral temporal lobectomy. The operation had spared the cortex, but destroyed the anterior two-thirds of the hippocampus, the amygdala, and the uncus bilaterally. Since the time of these observations, considerable agreement exists that in unilateral lobectomies, the side of the excision determines the kind of material that the individual will have trouble remembering: left-sided lesions being associated with impairments of memory for verbal material, right-sided lesions with nonverbal deficits. Further, the amount of the postoperative deficit seems related to the level of preoperation performance (Rausch, 1987), with patients demonstrating greater decreases with higher preoperative levels. There is a suggestion that improvements in memory function may occur for that memory type attributed to the temporal lobe contralateral to the one resected, especially for right-sided surgery (Rausch and Crandall, 1982). This is also reported following selective amygdalohippocampectomy, especially with good postoperative seizure control (Wieser, 1988).

Relationships between neuropathology and cognitive function were reported by Taylor (1981) and McMillan et al. (1987). In a complicated analysis, Taylor reported on gains and losses on IQ tests in 87 patients postoperatively. Noting that there are more patients for whom verbal IQ exceeds performance IQ for right-sided lesions (and the reverse for left resections), he did not notice that these biases were increased by operation. His data are shown in Table 7.1.

TABLE 7.1. *IQ Changes Following Temporal Lobectomy**

Group		P + V +	P − V −	P + V −	P − V +	Total
MTS	Left	5	2	0	1	8
	Right	4	1	0	3	8
AT	Left	1	1	7	0	9
	Right	4	4	1	0	9
Total		14	8	8	4	34
Both groups	Left	6	3	7	1	17
	Right	8	5	1	3	17

(Taylor, 1981)
*Gains or losses of verbal (V) and performance (P) IQ scores of 10 or more points on Wechsler tests following temporal lobectomy for epilepsy in 87 patients.

The results show few changes in the "lateralising" index in the P +, V − direction, and those present are largely confined to the removal of alien tissue lesions on the left side. Taylor's interpretation of this is that a left temporal lobe damaged by mesial temporal sclerosis has undergone a subsequent reorganization of functions, while a small left-sided alien tissue lesion has a more insidious effect within that lobe, still functioning preoperatively.

McMillan et al. (1987) reported on cognitive function before and at 4 weeks after temporal lobectomy. Hippocampal sclerosis was associated with poor preoperative intelligence and greater improvements across the operation compared with those with tumourlike malformations or nonspecific pathology. With regard to immediate verbal recall tasks, left-sided cases with other pathology had a poorer recall and right-sided patients had an above average recall, compared with no differences in the hippocampal sclerosis group. Postoperatively, scores for left temporal cases with other specific pathology had some impairments, right-sided cases having good immediate recall. Those with hippocampal sclerosis did not show apparent differences. Thus, changes across the operation were significant between pathological groups, revealing an improvement in other pathology cases and a slight worsening in hippocampal sclerosis cases. Similar results were given for a delayed verbal task, and there were no differences for nonverbal tasks.

These data, like those of Taylor, emphasise the potential importance of both the side of lesion and pathology in accounting for psychological deficits of patients before surgery, and the influence of temporal lobe resection on subsequent organisation of mental operations. Taylor also emphasises the importance of gender.

Psychiatric and Behavioural Results

The severe behaviour consequences of bilateral extirpation of the temporal lobes were soon realised, since several case studies or series were published in the early 1950s (Terzian, 1958). The operations, which included amygdalotomy, uncotomy, and medial temporal lobotomy were initially done for the relief of psychosis, mainly in schizophrenic patients, but some patients with epilepsy were included. Various elements of the Klüver-Bucy syndrome were reported, as were severe memory deficits, and the procedures gave way to unilateral operations.

In contrast to the recognised need for proper psychometric evaluation prior to surgery, the necessity for adequate psychiatric assessment has not been realised in many centres. The discrepancy emerged early in the history of these operations. Thus, the number of patients with preoperative psychiatric abnormalities was far greater in the Guy's-Maudsley series than in that from Montreal. This largely reflected referral patterns rather than a deliberate decision about the merits of operating on patients with behaviour problems. However, at some stage that Montreal group excluded patients with gross mental changes from operation (Hill et al., 1957). Further, in the early studies, it was agreed that some patterns of behaviour could change with temporal lobectomy, especially aggressive problems, while others were uninfluenced or deteriorated. Improvements were not immediate and could slowly occur over a period of 12 months or longer (Penfield, 1958). Green et al. (1951) were more explicit, noting that patients with constant hostility benefit from the operation, while those with psychotic behaviour do not.

The early experiences of Falconer and colleagues were written up in 1957 (Hill et al., 1957). Most of the 27 patients had resection of the anterior 6–8 cm of the temporal lobe including the uncus, hippocampus, and the amygdala, generally sparing the greater part of the superior temporal gyrus. All but one showed significant psychological disorder prior to surgery. Most had personality disorders rather than psychoses, the former largely referred to as character disorder (18). Two had an affective disorder, while the psychoses were paranoid in six and schizophrenic in one.

The postoperative follow-up was 2 to 5 years and included information from home visits, social work reports, parents, partners, employers, and others involved in the management of the patient. A rating scale comparing pre- to postoperative status was devised for work, sexuality, psychopathology, aggression, and need for hospitalization. Postoperative scores were improved in 18 cases, unchanged in 3, and declined in 5. All five of the latter continued to have seizures.

The specific changes reduced were aggression, with a "turning-in" of aggression. There was a reduction in outwardly turned aggressiveness which was replaced by depressive mood swings in 11 cases, the latter sometimes so severe that readmission to hospital was necessary, ECT being given to five. These depressive states tended to recur for up to 18 months and were not related to postoperative seizures. The authors comment: "The relation between inwardly turned aggressiveness and the depressive mental state, and outwardly turned aggressiveness and the hostile paranoid state is apparent in such patients. The postoperative personality changes of the temporal lobectomised patient would seem to create a 'model' psychosis susceptible for study because of its short duration, its intensity and its tendency to be altered by therapeutic measures" (Hill et al., 1957, p. 22).

A case is illustrated (Case 7.1), No. 25 of their series:

CASE 7.1

The patient was mildly paranoid prior to the week of operation, and remained quite unchanged until her discharge in the 8th postoperative week. From that time she became apathetic, seldom spoke, and frequently cried. She stated that she felt hopeless but was unable to give any depressive thought content. Punctuating this chronic state were aggressive outbursts of a florid paranoid type when she accused her mother and sister of talking about her in some derogatory way. She was unwilling to enlarge upon her ideas of references. She was admitted in an acutely depressed state 11 months after the operation but this fluctuated very rapidly . . . she was given three ECT which coincided with the disappearance of the depressive picture and an increase in the paranoid picture. She became so aggressive that this course of shock treatment was discontinued and by the time of her discharge three months later she showed neither depressive nor paranoid symptoms (Hill et al., 1957, p. 23).

In 14 patients there were changes in sexuality, which in general was of increased sexual drive and potency. One patient became hypersexual, while three lost "perverse sexual tendencies."

Other changes reported were of increased warmth in social relationships, increased extraversion, and a "lessening of egotism." The relationship of the psychosocial changes to seizure frequency was, in general, that those who became fit-free achieved a better level of adjustment.

Another early series was that of Simmel and Counts (1958) from Illinois. Forty patients were followed up after 5 years, and 11 were seizure-free. As with the Maudsley series, most patients had some personality disturbance or psychoses prior to surgery, although the extent of this is not well documented. They state "patients reported to talk about receiving messages from God, about their food being poisoned, etc., were classified as psychotic." Postoperative assessment was based on interviews with patients and their families, and patients were rated as "good," "marginal," or "psychotic."

Presurgery, 21 were marginal and 11 psychotic. At the time of follow-up, 19 were marginal and 14 psychotic. In terms of change, 2 were improved, 22 were about the same, while 16 deteriorated. Of the 14 psychotic patients, 10 were definitely psychotic before the operation, while 6 had "gone further downhill since surgery." It is of interest that of those who were said to have benefited, 4 were unchanged, 18 had right-sided operations and 6 left, while the deteriorated group had 7 right, 5 left, and 2 bilateral procedures. In summary, they note: "It does not appear to be true that anterior temporal lobectomy relieves patients with psychomotor epilepsy both of their seizures and their psychiatric difficulties. Nor is there any evidence that this operation makes the nonpsychotic patient psychotic. Rather, it seems that those patients who are not psychotic prior to surgery are more likely to benefit from the operation. . . . Patients who are psychotic before surgery continue to be so postoperatively, even if their seizures are improved, and in fact tend to deteriorate just as other psychotic patients do in the course of time" (Simmel and Counts, 1958, p. 537).

The above views were not totally supported by all of the surgeons involved with the early operations. For example, Falconer, discussing the paper of Simmel and Counts (1958) said: "The idea might get abroad that you cannot relieve such symptoms by temporal lobectomy . . . seven (of my psychiatric patients) had frank psychotic episodes, and three of them are now better . . . I feel at times psychiatric disturbances can be relieved in association with temporal lobectomies" (Falconer, 1958, pp. 557–558). Further, as noted below, the issue of the development of a postoperative psychosis *de novo* remains unsettled to this day.

Falconer (1973) specifically reviewed the consequences of temporal lobectomy on behaviour in an extended series of over 200 patients undergoing unilateral temporal lobectomy, followed up from 6 to 20 years. Nearly 50% of the cases had mesial temporal sclerosis; hamartomas accounted for a fifth to a quarter; a tenth had miscellaneous lesions such as scars or infarcts; no specific lesion was found in the rest. In a series of 100 cases (Serafetinides and Falconer, 1962), there were 12 with confusional states, 2 with sudden religious conversions, 6 were diagnosed as paranoid, and 3 were schizophrenic. Postoperatively there were two suicides, but of the remainder, six were said to be improved or recovered, and some working. Those with paranoid or affective conditions preoperatively had less prominent delusions postoperatively, while the schizophrenia group did poorly. Patients in a third group with intermittent symptoms, often ictally linked, did rather better.

Falconer noted an association between hamartomas and psychosis, especially for a schizophrenia-like presentation. This theme was taken up by Taylor in studies described below in a second series of 100 patients in which there were 16 cases of psychosis before operation, continuing in 12 postoperatively. He cited a remarkable case of a female operated on at the age of $2^{1}/_{2}$ years, free of seizures since the procedure, who at the age of 17 developed schizophrenia.

Falconer also reported on aggressive behaviour. Preoperatively, aggressive behaviour was as common with mesial temporal sclerosis as with hamartomas, but postoperatively, patients with mesial temporal sclerosis improved the most. In general, his data show that aggression is more likely associated with the male sex, early onset epilepsy, and a left-sided lesion.

Some of these cases were in the series reported by Glithero and Slater (1963). They reported 11 cases of schizophrenia-like psychosis and epilepsy. Their results are shown in Table 7.2. The schizophrenic symptoms had receded in only three, but in another five they were reported as improved.

In a series of papers, Taylor evaluated the relationship between epilepsy and psychosis using Falconer's cases (Taylor and Falconer, 1968; Taylor, 1975). In the first report on 100 cases, the mean length of follow-up was 68 months. Only 13 were considered psychiatrically normal before the operation. On a social adjustment scale, 61% were reported as improved, 28% worse, and 11% the same when pre- and postoperative scores were compared. It is of interest that five patients had committed suicide. In terms of "good," that is, clinically useful change, there were 51 patients with good postoperative adjustment compared with 34 before operation, an increase of 17. The main improvements were in the areas of family and extra-familiar relationships and work status. Those patients with "good" postoperative

TABLE 7.2. *Follow-up Findings in 11 Temporal Lobectomy Patients*

Findings	Total
At home:	
Entirely	4
Mainly	5
Very little	2
Fits:	
None for 12 months	5
No problem	5
A serious problem	1
"Schizophrenia":	
Receded	3
Improved	5
No change	3
Organic changes:	
Present	6
Absent	5

(Glithero and Slater, 1963)

adjustment showed an excess of normal or neurotic personalities prior to surgery, while those who fared worst had an excess of psychopathic disorder or psychoses. They also had a lower incidence of mesial temporal sclerosis and an increase in nonspecific lesions on pathological examination of the resected specimen.

Specifically with regard to psychosis, it was reported that only three patients who were rated psychotic postoperatively had mesial temporal sclerosis, whereas nine would have been expected by chance. Finally, complete relief of seizures was not essential for good adjustment, but 60% of those who moved from "bad" to "good" social adjustment with the operation became seizure-free.

In a later paper, Taylor (1975) considered in detail the factors that were associated with the schizophrenia-like psychoses in this selected surgical population. Forty-one patients with mesial temporal sclerosis were compared with 47 with "alien tissue" lesions, which included small tumours, hamartomas, and focal dysplasias. The diagnosis of schizophrenia-like psychosis was based upon findings at the time of the operation, or at follow-up interview. He noted that the psychotic symptoms were often subtle, and while florid schizophrenic symptoms were generally absent, paranoid ideas, fixed ideas, and incongruity of affect were the most evident.

In the total sample of 88, 13 were psychotic. There were 47 right-sided and 41 left-sided operations. The interactions between pathology, age of onset, gender, handedness, side of operation, and presence or absence of psychosis are shown in Figure 7.2. Of patients in the alien tissue group, 23% were psychotic compared with 5% with mesial temporal sclerosis. The psychosis was more frequent in left-sided compared with right-sided operations (22% and 9%), and in females (24%) compared with males (9%). There was a significant interaction between left-handedness and psychosis, as there was between left-handedness and alien tissue lesions.

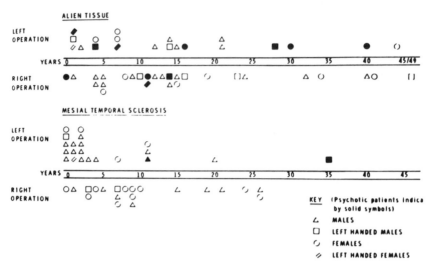

FIG. 7.2. Relationship between age of onset of epilepsy, psychosis, handedness, and pathology in patients with and without psychosis, from the data of Taylor (1975). (Reproduced with permission.)

Taylor's conclusion was that psychosis did not occur at random in patients with temporal lobe epilepsy, and he suggested that left-handed females with alien tissue lesions were most at risk and that left hemisphere lesions carried a greater risk than right-sided ones. This led to speculations regarding the differing role of the cerebral hemispheres in development and the influence of pathological lesions operating on different sexes at different times of life. Mesial temporal sclerosis derives from a postnatal insult while many of the alien tissue lesions are embryonic in origin, although most patients with the latter pathology had their first fit after the age of ten. Male and female brains develop differently, the vulnerability of the left brain to develop mesial temporal sclerosis being of longer duration in males than females. Since females with left alien tissue lesions seem the most vulnerable, Taylor argues that perhaps males with equivalent lesions have severe disorders that preclude surgery. Mesial temporal sclerosis damages the temporal lobe widely, while alien tissue lesions occupy a variety of positions in the temporal lobe. He noted: "Perhaps it is better, from the point of view of avoiding psychosis, that the lobe be nonfunctional rather than dysfunctional" (Taylor, 1975, p. 253).

In another follow-up study, Taylor and Marsh (1977) examined postoperative deaths in 193 temporal lobectomy patients who had a potential survival of at least 5 years. Four patients died from tumours, seven from natural causes, eight in status, and three in accidents. There were nine suicides and six deaths in "unclear" circumstances. The interval between operation and death was shorter in those who committed suicide or whose mode of death was unclear compared with the rest. Interestingly, the mortality in the first 2 years postoperatively was double that in any subsequent 2-year period.

The Maudsley series has recently been the subject of another follow-up investigation reported by Bruton (1988). He examined the notes and pathological specimens from 249 cases operated on from 1950. He assessed fit frequency and social adjustment, both graded into four categories ranging from greatly improved to worse. The former included only those fit-free for 5 years, and the social adjustment was based on such items as return to work, subsequent marriage, living away from institutional care; special attention was given to depression, aggression, and schizophrenia.

Of 27 deaths, there were 6 suicides which occurred at an average of 5.6 years after the operation. The results of surgery on personality and social adjustment in 234 cases revealed 59 to be greatly improved, 53 improved, 73 unaltered, and 49 worse. Thus, 48% benefited, 52% remained the same or deteriorated. Again it was found that the Ammon's horn sclerosis group had the best chance of improvement, while those with no abnormality were made significantly worse by the operation. The relationship between psychopathology and neuropathology is shown in Table 7.3.

This shows a substantial increase in depression, especially in those with Ammon's horn sclerosis, double pathology, and no apparent pathology. All 6 suicides were in this series of 24, but not associated with any clear pathology. Aggression clearly improves in both the alien tissue and the Ammon's horn sclerosis groups, while the frequency of schizophrenia-like psychosis alters little, but the distribution of the cases altered, especially if the alien tissue pathology was considered.

The data on the associations between psychosis and pathology have been reported in more detail by Roberts et al. (1990). In the total series, 25 patients had either pre- or a postoperative case note diagnoses of schizophrenia. The diagnosis in relation to the pathology is given in Table 7.4. Of 16 with a preoperative diagnosis of schizophrenia, 11 had a left- and 5 a right-sided focus. Postoperatively the figures were 5 and 4, respectively. In all cases where the lesion was localised, it was in the medial temporal structures; in 40% of cases the pathology was Ammon's horn sclerosis, this being found in 49% of the entire series. However, in contrast to the left/right distribution of the whole sample being equal (54 and 53 cases, respectively), the

TABLE 7.3. *Psychopathology and Neuropathology in Temporal Lobectomy Patients*

Pathology	Depression		Aggression		Schizophrenia	
	Preop	Postop	Preop	Postop	Preop	Postop
Development	0	1	1	1	1	0
Alien tissue	0	1	10	5	3	3
Ammon's horn Sclerosis	0	7	32	16	6	7
Inflammatory	0	0	2	2	0	0
Indefinite	0	2	1	2	1	1
No apparent pathology	1	9	6	7	4	5
Double pathology	0	4	2	2	0	2
Trauma	0	0	2	2	0	0
Total (% of Total)	1 (0.4%)	24 (10%)	56 (22%)	37 (16%)	15 (6%)	18 (7%)

(Bruton, 1988)

TABLE 7.4. *Incidence of Schizophrenia According to Neuropathological Group*

Pathological group	Side of focus	No.	Preoperative schizophrenic	Postoperative schizophrenic
Developmental	L	4	1	—
	R	2	—	—
Trauma	L	4	—	—
	R	6	—	—
A.T. Astrocytic	L	6	1	—
	R	3	—	—
A.T. Ganglioglial	L	3	—	1
	R	6	—	3
A.T. Cortical Dysplasia	L	5	—	—
	R	3	—	—
A.T. Oligodendrocytic	L	4	—	—
	R	2	—	—
A.T. Mixed Glial	L	5	—	1
	R	8	1	—
A.T. Vascular	L	2	—	—
	R	2	—	—
AHS	L	54	6	2
	R	53	2	—
Inflammatory	L	5	—	—
	R	6	—	—
Indefinite	L	11	—	—
	R	14	1	1
No Lesion	L	25	3	—
	R	16	1	1

(Roberts et al., 1990)

distribution of the lesions in the psychotic patients was significantly different, with eight left- and two right-sided resections. Patients with alien tissue or no lesions accounted for 20% of the psychotic cases, and the proportion of cases with alien tissue gangliogliomas who developed psychosis was significantly greater than expected. Further, there were four patients who lost their psychosis after the operation: three with Ammon's horn sclerosis and one with alien tissue, all being left-sided lobectomies. Birth injury, head injury, and febrile convulsions were present to the same degree in both psychotic and nonpsychotic patients.

There are several important conclusions that emerge from these data. First, in agreement with Taylor, it seems that schizophrenia-like states do not emerge at random in temporal lobe epilepsy. They are associated with medial temporal pathology but not exclusively with alien tissue lesions, as Taylor suggested. Bruton makes the point, however, that both Ammon's horn sclerosis and gangliogliomas lead to early onset seizures in their series (5.2 and 6.4 years, respectively), as opposed to middle and late teens for other pathologies. Second, there is an overrepresentation of left-sided pathology, as noted by Taylor, but the relationship holds only for assessment preoperatively. Bruton reported on nine cases that became psychotic postoperatively, in whom five had right lobectomies, but interestingly, all cases that appeared to lose their psychosis had undergone left lobectomies. Postoperative status thus reflects a bias toward right-sided lesions, increasing the vulnerability to develop a psychosis, left-sided lesions favouring amelioration. Third, ganglioglial lesions may have a special relationship to psychosis. The pathological picture is essentially that of a mixed glial abnormality, with the addition of abnormal, often giant, nerve cells resembling ganglion cells scattered throughout the lesion. They are often calcified and in some cases are associated with Ammon's horn sclerosis. They lead to early onset seizures, and in Bruton's series, their removal, while leading to a good result as far as seizure control is concerned, did not improve social adjustment, and four developed a schizophrenia-like psychosis. Roberts et al. (1990) point out that the neuronal elements in these tumours have synaptic contacts with other neurones and potentially could disrupt signal transmission in temporal structures, especially at crucial times of development.

Finally, Bruton's data reveal the dissociation between the effect of temporal lobectomy on seizures and on behavioural adaptation. It is often assumed that a decrease of seizures is automatically associated with improved behaviour, but this is not the case. His league table of benefits and costs is given in Table 7.5. It emphasises the importance of the underlying pathology, and the fact that the best overall results are seen with Ammon's horn sclerosis.

TABLE 7.5. *Effects of Surgery: League Table of Benefits** *

Diagnostic groups	No. of patients in group	% of total sample	Comments
Ammon's horn sclerosis	107	43.0	Benefit: both fit frequency and social adjustment
Mixed glial	9	3.6	Benefit: fits only. Social adjustment unaffected
Neuronoglial (ganglioglial)	5	3.0	Benefit: fits only. Social adjustment unaffected
Astrocytic	8	3.2	Unaffected
Oligodendrocytic	5	2.0	Unaffected
Neuronoglial (cortical dysplasia)	8	3.2	Unaffected
Vascular	3	1.2	Unaffected
Developmental lesion	5	2.0	Unaffected
Inflammatory	8	3.2	Unaffected
Double pathology	18	7.3	Unaffected
Trauma	7	2.8	Fits unaffected. Social adjustment worse
Indefinite pathology	25	10.0	Fits unaffected. Social adjustment worse
No apparent abnormality	41	16.5	Fits unaffected. Social adjustment worse

(Bruton, 1988)
*Temporal lobectomy series: 249 patients.

TABLE 7.6. *Psychiatric Status Following Temporal Lobectomy*

	Denmark Copenhagen	England Guy's-M.	France Marseilles	U.S.S.R. Sverdlovsk	USA UI Chicago	Total
Surviving patients	72	72	50	69	60	323
% Normal before and after	8.3	9.7	—	—	} 11.7	} 23.5
% Normalized	22.2	25.0	} 52.0	31.9		
% Markedly improved	27.8	31.9		} 37.7	3.3	} 40.9
% Improved	6.9	18.1			28.3	
% Unchanged/ deteriorated	34.7	15.3	48.0	30.4	56.6	35.6

(Jensen, 1975)

Although most follow-up studies have been carried out on the Maudsley series, other centres have also provided data. The state of the art in 1975 was noted in the review by Jensen. Table 7.6 is taken from her paper and shows the follow-up psychiatric status from five centres, including the Maudsley.

There is a marked divergence of results, especially with regard to the "unchanged/deteriorated" category; this may reflect on selection or on the adequacy of the evaluations. Jensen noted that, on summing the different series, 23.5% were considered mentally normal at the time of follow-up, compared with 6.2% before operation. In contrast, 35% were unchanged or deteriorated.

Further data from the Danish series were given by Jensen and colleagues, especially with regard to psychosis (Jensen and Vaernet, 1977; Jensen and Larsen, 1979a; 1979b). They surveyed 74 patients who had received unilateral temporal lobectomy, 45 (61%) of whom were seizure-free postoperatively. Prior to operation, 85% were rated as psychiatrically abnormal and 11 were psychotic, all with paranoid delusions. The abnormalities are shown in Table 7.7.

The behavioural disturbances ranged from hyperactivity to severe aggression, and the miscellaneous category included dementia, reactions of self-reference and paranoid temper, and episodes of dysphoria. The predominant sexual disturbance was lack of libido, noted in 31%.

After surgery, 5 patients previously judged mentally well became psychiatrically ill, and 16 with psychiatric symptoms improved. All suicide attempts occurred within the first postoperative month.

TABLE 7.7. *Types of Psychiatric Abnormality from the Danish Series*

	Preoperative	Postoperative
Psychosis	11	20
Suicidal attempt	11	6
Behavioural disturbance	54	33
Sexual aggression	4	5
Neurosis	7	5
Drugs or alcohol abuse	27	29
One or more of above	63 (85.1%)	50 (69.4%)

(Jensen and Vaernet, 1977)

Relief of seizures was the most important factor in determining rehabilitation to work, but there was no obvious relationship between postoperative seizure frequency and psychiatric status. Behavioural disturbances were the most improved by operation, a finding in keeping with other series.

In Jensen's series there were 20 psychotic patients, either pre- or postoperatively. Seventeen had partial seizures with secondary generalization. Eleven were psychotic preoperatively, and one recovered after surgery. Nine patients became psychotic postoperatively, and in six there was complete relief of seizures. The 20 cases were divided into three main groups: schizophrenia-like states (13), paranoid delusions and depression (6), and chronic psychosis dominated by autism (1). Of this total sample, ten cases had the schizophrenia-like psychosis described by Slater and colleagues (1963) (see Chapter 8).

Statistically significant associations were found between focal neuropathological lesions and psychosis (11 of 20), and a higher frequency of major psychiatric disorder was recorded in near relatives (65% compared with 39% in nonpsychotic patients). Further, psychotic patients had been more often the subject of perinatal complications.

Eight of the eleven cases with preoperative psychosis improved with surgery, although to what degree is not stated. Curiously, the important issue of laterality is glossed over by the statement that "operations on the right or on the nondominant sides were more frequent in the psychotic patients," but no figures were given. This series is of importance in confirming that psychosis can arise *de novo* postoperatively and that this is seen in spite of, or because of, seizure relief. One speculation which emerges is that, at least in some of these cases, a mechanism similar to that of forced normalisation is operative.

Other groups have provided limited information on the behavioural changes of patients undergoing temporal lobectomy. Sherwin (1981), in a study of patients with psychosis who had undergone lobectomy, noted seven cases rendered seizure-free in whom no change in psychosis was observed. Walker and Blumer (1984) provided data on 50 patients. Irritability, anger, and rage noted in 29 patients preoperatively improved in 22, although 6 patients developed such behaviours. There were nine psychotic patients, one case of which was alcohol-related. Six patients developed a schizophrenia-like psychosis postoperatively, this developing some time after the operation in three. No data on pathology or laterality were given, and the general conclusion drawn was that temporal lobectomy had little or no effect on psychosis associated with epilepsy.

Stevens (1991) followed a personal series of 14 patients for 25 to 30 years, six of whom were psychiatrically well, five being seizure-free. However, six became psychiatrically worse postoperatively, three of whom were reported as normal before surgery. No less than five developed a paranoid psychosis, four of whom had right-sided operations. The majority were not seizure-free.

Polkey (1983) has given data on a new Maudsley series of 40 patients, 17 of whom had some form of mental disorder preoperatively. Aggression was the most common, and there were no psychotic patients. Postoperatively two developed psychosis, and Polkey describes a third not in the series of 40. All had nondominant resections, and in one who subsequently died in an accident the opposite temporal lobe was pathologically normal. In another, the psychosis resolved when the patient's seizures returned.

Several groups have used some form of objective rating scale to assess patients postoperatively. Meier and French (1965) found some changes on the MMPI at follow-up of 1 year or more, especially paranoia. No differences between right- and left-sided operations were noted. Cairns (1974) reported no change using the 16 Personality Factor Questionnaire of Cattell and the Hostility and Direction of Hostility Questionnaire of Foulds. This study did not refer to the more severe and psychotic aspects of behaviour. Wieser (1988) used the Bear-Fedio Personality Inventory in 42 patients who had received amygdalohippocampectomy. The data are shown in Fig. 7.3. Patients who were rendered seizure-free had the lowest scores, those unchanged showing high scores on some psychotic subscales such as paranoia.

CONCLUSIONS

These data on the psychiatric consequences of temporal lobectomy lead to several conclusions. First, most centres, including the Maudsley hospital group, have now stopped operating on floridly psychotic patients. This seems largely based on the observation that psychosis generally does not improve with the operation (Serafetinides and Falconer, 1962; Jensen and Larsen, 1979a, 1979b). Whether or not this is justified is not clear in the sense that it might still be considered better to be psychotic without seizures than to be psychotic with them. This policy, however, has not been taken to its logical conclusion, namely, that of a comprehensive psychiatric evaluation being carried out preoperatively. This is in marked contrast to the insistence, correctly, on good psychological assessment.

It seems that the psychosocial adjustment of patients postoperatively is by no means as good as the results on seizures, and in some series as many patients deteriorate as improve. The improvements in behaviour generally recorded are those of aggression, irritability, and disturbed conduct, and these seem more likely to improve with improvement of seizures. In contrast, postoperative depression and both early and late suicide are reported from several groups, which may be seen as a complication of the surgery. Some authors suggest this may be no more than a reflection of the high frequency of depression in nonoperated epileptic patients. The figure of 10% of patients developing depression, and the six suicides, given by Bruton (1988) nonetheless emphasise the need for continuing psychiatric observation of operated patients. This is not done in most centres. Indeed, the number of good follow-up series of psychiatric data, considering the number of centres now doing such procedures, is abysmal.

It is also clear that a psychosis, paranoid or schizophrenia-like in nature, may develop *de novo* postoperatively, and the frequency of this in each series is given in

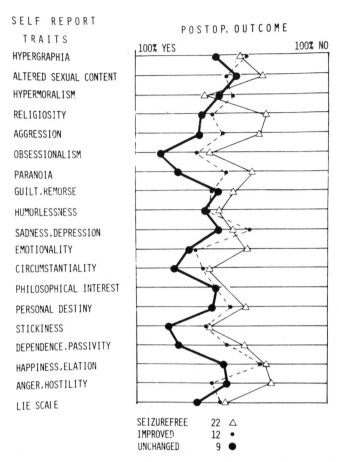

FIG. 7.3. Postoperative personality profiles of patients following selective amygdalohippocampectomy. (From Weiser, 1988, with permission.)

Table 7.8. This gives a mean figure of 7.4% of 456 cases, ranging from 3.8% to 28.5%. Again this emphasises the importance of postoperative behavioural assessments and continuing supervision of patients. There are no clear predictors of the patients who will develop the psychoses; neither is there agreement as to the relationship to the seizure control. There is, nonetheless, the suggestion that the phenomenon of forced normalisation may be operative in at least some cases. Again it could be argued that the patients would have gone on to develop psychoses in any case, as is suggested in the remarkable patient of Taylor's who developed psychosis so many years after an operation in early childhood. This difficulty is emphasised in case 6.1, in which the patient with an ictally related psychosis postoperatively developed a hebephrenia with marked deterioration. This could have perhaps been expected from the natural history of schizophrenia except this patient had an epi-

TABLE 7.8. *Postoperative Psychosis: New Cases*

	Total	Psychosis (%)	Laterality*
Simmel and Counts, 1958	44	4 (9)	1R, 2L, 1B
Jensen and Larsen, 1979a,b	74	9 (12.1)	data unavailable
Polkey, 1983	40	2 (5)	2R
Walker and Blumer, 1984	50	6 (12)	data unavailable
Bruton, 1988	234	9 (3.8)	5R
Stevens, 1991	14	4 (28.5)	4R
Total:	456	34 (7.4)	

*(L) Left, (R) Right, (B) Bilateral

lepsy-related psychosis. Such patients tend not to deteriorate over time (see Chapter 9). The argument is supported by the high genetic loading for psychiatric illness in the series of Jensen and Larsen (1979b), this aspect not being commented on by other authors.

Another explanation was given by Ferguson and Rayport (1965). They described five patients whose behaviour deteriorated after lobectomy, in spite of seizures improving and the EEG being normal in three. As in the case described by Polkey (1983), one patient improved when seizures returned. The authors suggested that the seizures had some "ego-syntonic" function for patients, quoting Freud with approval: "The epileptic discharge places itself at the disposal of the neurosis, the essence of which is to get rid by somatic means of masses of stimuli which it can not deal with physically" (Freud, 1953). Ferguson and Rayport (1965) thus say: "The illness often shields the patient from the fuller expression of the sterner feelings he arouses in his ambivalent environment . . . the illness may cause recognition to be bestowed despite inadequacy of performance and may shield the patient from day-to-day demands or obligations" (p. 33). For them, rehabilitation is reversed in this setting, and instead of having to get the patient to learn to live with his handicap, he must learn to live without it.

A remarkable finding emerges from a consideration of the new cases of psychosis (see Table 7.8), which suggests that such a sociological explanation is insufficient to explain more severe psychopathology, especially the psychoses. Where laterality has been established, it is right-sided in over 60% of cases, rising to 73% if the very early series is omitted. Bruton even suggested a link to a specific pathology, namely gangliogliomas. This overrepresentation of right-sided operations is supported further by the series of Mace and Trimble (1991), in which six consecutive cases are described; all developed postoperative psychoses; all had right-sided operations.

The best results from the point of view of psychiatric status, especially in antisocial and aggressive behaviours, results from removal of mesial temporal sclerosis. This lesion is associated with psychosis, and the earlier contention of Taylor that schizophrenia-like psychosis is almost exclusively associated with hamartomas was not supported, for example, by the study of Jensen and Larsen (1979a, 1979b). Of their 13 patients with this type of psychosis, only 4 had such pathological lesions.

8

Interictal Psychosis

In Chapter 1 the development of the concept that behavioural disturbances of epilepsy could be manifested outside the ictal period was traced. Many of the early authors (see below) discussed the development of psychotic states, case histories being provided which would be recognisable and classifiable in today's terminology. It was noted how, in the early part of this century, the concept of an antagonism between psychotic states and epileptic seizures arose, and in Chapter 5 these ideas were fully explored, noting how an increased association between epilepsy and psychosis was compatible with an antagonistic relationship between the symptoms of psychosis and seizures.

Examples of ictally related psychoses were discussed in Chapter 6, and there can be few physicians managing patients with chronic epilepsy who have not seen such states. The issue of psychosis interictally, however, occasions considerable controversy, and much of this is explored in this and in the following chapter. In order to fully understand the development of concepts related to these arguments and to explore further the relationship between psychotic symptoms and epilepsy, it is necessary to briefly review an even more controversial area, namely, the association between epilepsy and personality disorder.

PERSONALITY DISORDER

The history of the relationship between epilepsy and personality was summarised by Guerrant et al. (1962). The "period of epileptic deterioration," typifying views in the last half of the last century, implied that personality deterioration was a consequence of the disease itself, or possibly as a sequel to prolonged use of bromide therapy. Around the turn of the century, the term *epileptic character*, introduced originally by Morel, acquired a specific meaning, and concepts regarding its development became intertwined with Freudian psychodynamics. Turner (1907) provided an early example of the change:

> In early days the convulsion, or fit, was regarded as the sole element of importance in the clinical study of epilepsy; but in more recent years the psychical factor has come to

be looked upon as of almost equal importance, and both are regarded as manifestations of a predisposition associated with inheritance. . . . it is rare to find epileptics who do not present some form of mental obliquity . . . the possession of which is a feature of their hereditarily degenerative disposition. . . . the mental condition is not solely a consequence of seizures but is an expression of the same nervous constitution which gives rise to the convulsion (p. 2).

The belief was that epilepsy was a constitutional disorder in which the seizures were but one manifestation of more diverse symptomatology. The psychoanalytic expression of this was most forcefully put by Clark (1923), who recognised pre-epileptic constitutions, suggesting that the seizure itself was simply a psychological regressive and protective mechanism employed by an overstressed ego.

At the time such theories were being put forward, there were many writers who acknowledged that some patients with epilepsy may show psychiatric difficulties, but by and large reported that their patients were normal from the psychological point of view. Lennox forcefully made the point in a review of personality in epilepsy, suggesting that the majority of patients with epilepsy were entirely normal and that difficulties which arose were related to complex interactions between the various complications of having epilepsy. These included, for example, anoxia, or cerebral damage with repeated seizures, the prolonged administration of anticonvulsant drugs, and disabling psychological reactions to social stigmatism which was so common in epilepsy (Lennox and Lennox, 1960).

The introduction of the EEG into clinical practice and the clear delineation of a type of epilepsy deriving from the temporal lobes led to what Guerrant et al. (1962) have referred to as the "period of psychomotor peculiarity." The two groups most influential in developing these ideas were those of Gibbs and colleagues from the United States and Gastaut and collaborators in France.

The views of the former school may be best summarised by the quotation of Gibbs and Stamps (1953) that: "The patient's emotional reactions to his seizures, his family and to his social situation are less important determinants of psychiatric disorder than the site and type of the epileptic discharge" (p. 78).

Gibbs (1951) noted that anterior temporal foci were common in epileptic patients, and further that the highest instance of psychiatric disorder occurred in cases with a spike focus in this region. Figure 8.1, taken from Gibbs (1951), shows the percentage of severe personality disorder and psychosis associated with various sites of epileptic focus.

Gibbs made the important statement that the psychiatric symptoms accompanying psychomotor epilepsy were indistinguishable from those encountered in "purely psychiatric disorders," and suggested that pathological and physiological involvement of temporal lobe structures were related to their presentation.

Gastaut and his group clearly documented the underlying neuropathological changes of psychomotor seizures, reemphasising the importance of Ammon's horn sclerosis. They also identified an association between behaviour disorders and seizures which arise from medial temporal structures. In one of the earliest controlled studies of personality in epilepsy, Gastaut et al. (1953) compared 43 patients with

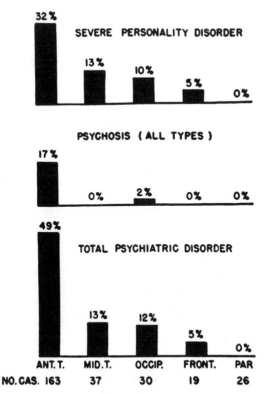

FIG. 8.1. The incidence of psychopathology in patients with various sites of epileptic abnormality (Gibbs, 1951).

psychomotor epilepsy to 21 suffering from generalised functional epilepsy and a smaller group with symptomatic epilepsy with neocortical surface lesions. Only patients with lesions involving limbic structures, the majority of whom had psychomotor seizures and temporal lobe EEG abnormalities, showed personality disorders.

In discussion of this area, much confusion has arisen due to a misunderstanding of the history outlined above. In particular, two concepts have become confused; namely, the ideas stemming from the era of psychosomatic medicine postulating susceptible personalities (the period of the "epileptic character"), and the later ideas of "psychomotor peculiarity." The latter essentially emphasise that patients with chronic lesions in temporal structures (limbic system in particular) could go on to develop secondary personality disorders. The precedent for this had been set by the clear delineation of frontal lobe personality changes and the discovery of behavioural changes in animals following bilateral lesions of the amygdala in the Klüver-Bucy syndrome.

Tizard (1962) critically reviewed the concept of the epileptic personality in studies which had been carried out up to 1962. She pointed out the major methodological difficulties including selection bias, assessment reliability and validity, and the large number of studies that had relied on Rorschach testing, notorious for the subjective nature of its interpretation. Since that review, a number of studies have been carried out, some of which have attempted to specifically answer these criticisms, including that of Guerrant et al. (1962). These are summarised in Tables 8.1 and 8.3.

In this table, only adult studies that have used some form of rating scale have

TABLE 8.1. *Personality and Epilepsy: Adult Studies Since 1962**

Author	Number of cases	Result
Guerrant et al., 1962	32 TLE 26 Primary GEN 26 Chronic medical illness	All groups similar: medical illness—more neurosis GEN—more Pd; TLE—more psychosis.
Small et al., 1962	25 Psychomotor 25 Centrencephalic or extratemporal foci	No differences: high scores both groups.
Kløve and Doehring, 1962	20 Epilepsy, unknown aetiology 20 Symptomatic epilepsy 20 Brain damage, no epilepsy 20 Affective disturbances 20 Controls	Epilepsy of unknown aetiology highest scores.
Meier and French, 1965	53 TLE	Bilateral > unilateral esp validity,D,Pa, Sc, caudality Independent > dependent.
Matthews and Kløve, 1968	51 Nonneurological controls 48 Brain damage, no epilepsy 65 Epilepsy, known aetiology (23 major motor; 22 psychomotor; 20 mixed) 69 Epilepsy, unknown aetiology: (29 major motor, 22 Psychomotor, 18 mixed)	No differences. D most frequently elevated in epileptic patients. Most abnormalities in nonneurological controls.
Mignone et al., 1970	98 Psychomotor 53 Nonpsychomotor	No differences between psychomotor and nonpsychomotor. Sc increased in those psychomotor with generalised seizures. Deviant responses: dominant > nondominant.
Stevens et al., 1972	29 Psychomotor 14 Generalised 6 Focal	No differences. Sc scale—high scores for psychomotor and generalised.
Rodin et al., 1976	78 TLE 78 Controls	TLE higher on D and Pa.
Lachar et al., 1979	37 TLE 28 Non-TLE	None
Hermann et al., 1980	47 TLE	Adolescent onset associates with increased ppd, Pt, Sc, Pa compared with child and adult onset.

TABLE 8.1. *Continued*

Author	Number of cases	Result
Hermann et al., 1982a	TLE Ictal fear 11 Other aura 14 generalised 16	Ictal fear higher than other on psychopathic deviate, Pa, Pt, Sc, Social introversion Goldbergs system generalised—normal TLE—other aura, abnormal neurotic TLE—fear, abnormal psychotic.
Hermann et al., 1982b	33 complex partial seizures 34 complex partial seizures with secondary GEN	complex partial seizures with 2 generalisation score higher.
Dikmen et al., 1983	37 complex partial seizures 25 secondary generalised 34 complex partial seizures with generalisation 48 Primary generalised	complex partial seizures with 2 GEN higher D

*MMPI Scale; (Ca) Caudality, (CPS) complex partial seizures, (D) depression, (F) validity, (GEN) generalised, (N) neurosis, (P) psychosis, (Pa) paranoia, (Pd) personality disturbance, (ppd) psychopathic deviate, (Pt) psychasthenia, (Sc) schizophrenia, (Si) Social introversion, (TLE) temporal lobe epilepsy.

been included, and in the majority of studies some attempt has been made to compare patients with either temporal lobe or psychomotor epilepsy with epilepsy of some other form.

MMPI STUDIES

Considering the MMPI studies, 13 are quoted and several conclusions emerge. First, the earlier studies fail to show significant differences between temporal lobe epilepsy or its variants and other form of seizures. However some of the studies are complicated in that nonepileptic control groups also score high on psychopathology (Guerrant et al., 1962; Matthews and Kløve, 1968), or alternative psychological tests suggest that "centrencephalic" or generalised seizure patients have more cerebral damage than one would suspect from a primary generalised seizure disorder; for example, patients doing worse on psychological tests than those in the psychomotor group (Small et al., 1962; Stevens et al., 1972). Second, some differences do emerge, especially in subcatagories of patients with temporal lobe disorder. Bilateral findings appear to provoke more disturbances of personality than unilateral lesions (Meier and French, 1965) while those with multiple seizure types or secondarily generalised seizures also score more deviant profiles (Mignone et al., 1970, Rodin et al., 1976; Hermann et al., 1982b).

Rodin et al. (1976) explored this in most detail, comparing patients with temporal lobe seizures and one seizure type with those with more than one seizure type, and then comparing control patients who have one seizure type with those who have more than one seizure type. The first analysis revealed higher elevation of MMPI scores in patients with more than one seizure type, while the second evaluation did not. In other words, behavioural abnormalities did not increase solely as the result of having more than one seizure type, and was overrepresented in the temporal lobe population. A third analysis, comparing patients with temporal lobe epilepsy and more than one seizure type to controls with more than one seizure type, was also performed. The temporal lobe group showed more psychotic tendencies and higher elevation of paranoia on the MMPI. A problem in interpretation of such comparisons is that patients with temporal lobe epilepsy, generally, as shown in the Rodin et al. (1976) study, are prescribed more anticonvulsants, tend to have more clusters of seizures, and more frequently have a known aetiology for their attacks.

Third, the scales which tend to be reported abnormal most frequently when differences are noted are the depression scale (D); the paranoia scale (Pa), representing suspiciousness, oversensitivity, ideas of references and delusions of persecution; the schizophrenia scale (Sc) representing behaviour characterised by bizarre and unusual thoughts; and the psychasthenia (Pt) scale, which is related to classifications of phobia or obsessive-compulsive behaviour. The relevance of this for the understanding of psychosis is that several of these scales directly record psychotic symptomatology, and these are the ones which are most often noted to be abnormal.

Finally, some of the later studies have selected out subgroups of patients who appear to be particularly susceptible to the development of these changes, especially towards the psychotic dimension. For example, the association of adolescent age of onset with a higher frequency of reporting of these psychotic subscales (Hermann et al., 1980), although this was not found in the study of Mignone et al. (1970) when they viewed their overall sample of patients. Further, the finding of Hermann et al. (1982a), that patients with an aura of ictal fear are more susceptible to record high scores on the MMPI profiles, especially paranoia, psychasthenia, schizophrenia, and psychopathic deviation (represented by absence of deep emotional responses and meaningful interpersonal relationships), is one of a series of studies (Table 8.2) in which the suggestion that not all patients with temporal lobe epilepsy will be susceptible to psychopathology, but only a subgroup with medial temporal or limbic seizures is explored (see below).

The MMPI studies have been subject to a metanalysis by Whitman et al. (1984). They used Goldberg's (1972) sequential diagnostic system which classifies from group MMPI profiles: normal or abnormal; if abnormal—sociopathic or psychiatric; if psychiatric—neurotic or psychotic. A total of 809 patients with epilepsy from 10 MMPI studies were compared with 1,107 patients from 15 MMPI studies with nonneurological illnesses. Further, there were 870 subjects from 22 MMPI studies with nonepileptic but neurological conditions. The latter included multiple sclerosis, cerebral palsy, and localised or diffuse brain damage. Their data revealed that patients with epilepsy were, as a group, at higher risk for psychopathology than the general population, although as a whole there was no evidence that people with epilepsy were at higher risk than patients with other chronic disorders. However, when neurotic and psychotic categorisation was studied, patients with epilepsy manifested more severe psychopathology than both the neurological or the illness control groups. Within the epilepsy group, however, there were no seizure differ-

TABLE 8.2. *Studies Showing More Psychopathology in Association with Medial Temporal/Limbic Seizures*

Author	Limbic flag	Scale	Changes
Kristensen and Sindrup,* 1978	Sphenoidal electrodes		Psychotic-epileptic patients more medio basal foci: abnormal-psychotic
Nielsen and Kristensen, 1981	EEG site of focus	BFI	Hypergraphia, elation, guilt and paranoia
Dana-Haeri et al., 1984	Neurohormones	Psychopathology	Greater release of prolactin in patients with psychopathology
Hermann et al., 1982a	Aura of fear	MMPI	Psychopathic deviate, paranoia, psychasthenia, schizophrenia, social introversion, abnormal psychotic
Wieser, 1983	Implanted electrodes	BFI	Neocortical vs. limbic: limbic score higher on hypergraphia, sex, humourlessness, sadness and philosophical interest
Stark-Adamec et al., 1985	Auras of: formed images humming jamais vu time changes	BFI	Seizure patients with psychopathology report more of these auras

*psychosis study

ences noted when temporal lobe epilepsy was compared with generalized epilepsy. Subgroups of patients with temporal lobe abnormalities were not, however, examined.

There has been a criticism that many of the MMPI studies are negative simply because the MMPI was not designed to assess psychopathology in epilepsy, and therefore would be an insensitive instrument. Dikmen et al. (1983) attempted to provide some evidence for the validity of the MMPI by comparing a group of patients with epilepsy who had a history of psychiatric difficulties and those with no such problems. The MMPI appeared sensitive to these changes, noting significant differences between the two groups on several scales. However, Dikmen et al. did criticise some of the earlier MMPI results, particularly the suggestion that the schizophrenia scale may be elevated more frequently in epileptic populations than would be expected. They pointed out that the 78 items on the MMPI Sc scale appear to describe the cognitive and dissociative sensory experiences which patients with epilepsy might be expected to report. Indeed, when they gave these items to board-certified neurologists, 37% of them were thought to be descriptive of seizure phenomena, anticonvulsant drug effects, or cognitive difficulties associated with brain damage.

In part to overcome some of the difficulties of interpretation of MMPI data, Bear and Fedio (1977) developed their own rating scale derived from prior reports of personality in epilepsy. They noted that many of the traits were not necessarily indicative of psychopathology, but were regularly referred to in the literature in relationship to interictal personality changes. Their data, and subsequent studies using this scale, in addition to the small number of other reports of personality in epilepsy are shown in Table 8.3.

NON-MMPI STUDIES

As with the MMPI studies, the results of investigations using the Bear-Fedio Inventory (BFI) are somewhat mixed (see Table 8.3). In their original report, Bear and Fedio (1977) compared patients with unilateral temporal lobe epilepsy to normal subjects and to a group having neuromuscular disorders. They noted that epileptic patients reported a different profile of responses to nonepileptic and controls, noting such personality features such as humourlessness, dependence, circumstantiality, increased sense of personal destiny, and others as being distinctive. There were differences between self-reported behaviour profiles and independent rater profiles from a close family member or friend. Laterality differences were noted: patients with left temporal epilepsy described more anger, paranoia, and dependence; while those with right temporal foci reported more elation. This group also examined MMPI profiles and noted no differences, emphasising the value of their new scale in temporal lobe epileptic patients.

Subsequent studies tended to either confirm or refute their findings, authors of the latter studies tending to imply that the scale did no more than assess nonspecific psychopathology (Mungas, 1982; Rodin and Schmaltz, 1984; Master et al., 1984). This was largely based on comparisons between patients hospitalised for psychiatric illness and patients with temporal lobe epilepsy, few or no differences being noted between these populations. While not supportive of a profile of psychopathology distinctive for temporal lobe epilepsy, these critics miss the point that there is a

TABLE 8.3. *Studies of Personality and Epilepsy—Non-MMPI*

Author	Scale	Number of cases	Result
Standage and Fenton, 1975	Present State Examination nonpsychotic: Eysenck Personality Inventory	27 Epilepsy 27 Medical controls	No difference— both groups high scores. TLE vs. non-TLE— no difference.
Bech et al., 1977	Marke-Nyman Inventory	30 Juvenile Myoclonic Epilepsy 29 Psychomotor 30 Grand mal 22 Controls (Ménière's)	Low validity in Juvenile Myoclonic Epilepsy.
Trimble and Perez, 1980	Middlesex Hosp Questionnaire	281 51% Generalised 36% TLE and generalised 8% TLE alone	No major difference.
Kogeorgos et al., 1982	General Health Questionnaire Crown-Crisp Experimental Index	66 Epilepsy 50 Neurological controls	No major difference.
Sorensen et al., 1988	Eysenck Personality Inventory Bellak Interview	28 TLE 15 Psoriasis 15 Primary GE 15 Controls	Ego functioning poorer in those with more than one seizure type. No R/L differences.
Bear and Fedio, 1977	BFI MMPI	27 TLE 15R 12L 12 Normal 9 Neuromuscular disorders	MMPI, no differences. BFI, many differences between TLE and others. R vs. L esp. paranoia, elation, dependence, anger.
Hermann and Riel, 1981	BFI	14 GE 14 CPS	TLE significantly greater on personal destiny, dependence, paranoia, philosophical interest.
Nielsen and Kristensen, 1981	BFI	Lateral focus 14-L 11-R Mediobasal focus 9-R 8-R	Mediobasal focus > lateral guilt and paranoia. L/R differences noted.

TABLE 8.3. *Continued*

Author	Scale	Number of cases	Result
Bear et al., 1982	BFI	10 TLE 10 other seizures 10 Affectives 10 Schizophrenia 10 Aggressive- ness	TLE and other seizures: TLE greater on religiosity, philosophical interests, sadness, emotionally and total test mean.
Mungas, 1982	BFI	14 TLE 14 Neurological and behavioural disorders 14 Psychiatric	No differences.
Rodin and Schmaltz, 1984	BFI	148 Epilepsy 16 RTLE 16 LTLE 18 Pain patients 15 Psychiatric 40 Controls	TLE scored higher in 13 categories, hypergraphia esp. No R/L differences. Relationship to anticonvulsant drugs.
Master et al., 1984	BFI	55 TLE 16 Primary GE 27 Psychiatric 40 Controls	No differences between patient groups. No R/L differences.
Brandt et al., 1985	BFI	28 LTLE 19 RTLE 10 Primary GE 14 Controls	LTLE and generalised patients most different from controls, esp. circumstantiality, humourlessness, sadness, viscosity, dependence, obsessionality, and paranoia.
Stark-Adamec et al., 1985	BFI	70 Seizure patients: CPS, GE, CPS+GE 92 Psychiatric 28 Dialysis 447 Nonpatients	Seizure patients do not differ from each other. Links of psychopathology in epilespy to auras.

(BFI) Bear-Fedio Inventory, (CPS) complex partial seizures, (GE) generalised epilepsy (L) left, (LTLE) left temporal lobe epilepsy, (MMPI) Minnesota Multiphasic Personality Inventory, (R) right, (RTLE) right temporal lobe epilepsy, (TLE) temporal lobe epilepsy.

cerebral basis to psychopathology in the absence of epilepsy, and that patients with conditions other than epilepsy may have disturbed function within their temporal lobes.

Of more interest are the positive findings; in regard to the relationship to psychosis a persistent reporting of paranoia in temporal lobe groups by four different studies is worthy of comment (Bear and Fedio, 1977; Hermann and Riel, 1981; Nielsen and Kristensen, 1981; Brandt et al., 1985). The studies hint at left temporal mediobasal abnormalities being the most relevant for this form of psychopathology.

Another trait which is distinguishing in several studies is that of hypergraphia (Bear and Fedio, 1977; Nielsen and Kristensen, 1981; Rodin and Schmaltz, 1984), which has become the subject of independent research studies (Figs. 8.2A and 8.2B) (Trimble, 1986). There is some evidence that this phenomenon may appear as an all-or-nothing state or trait in certain patients and is related to temporal lobe abnormalities, possibly of the nondominant hemisphere. Of more interest, however, is that the only other clinical group where hypergraphia is a recognised sign is in the major psychoses, namely, schizophrenia and mania.

A criticism of the BFI studies is that they have failed to confirm that all patients with temporal lobe epilepsy suffer from a distinctive personality profile which can be detected by the scale. While Bear and Fedio (1977) do refer to a consistent profile of changes noted in patients, it is not claimed that they would be seen in all patients at all times—clearly an unrealistic expectation.

The view that there is an interictal behaviour syndrome associated with temporal lobe epilepsy was, from the clinical point of view, most strongly supported by the writings of Geschwind and colleagues (Waxman and Geschwind, 1975). They highlighted changes in sexual behaviour, hypergraphia, and religiosity and provided

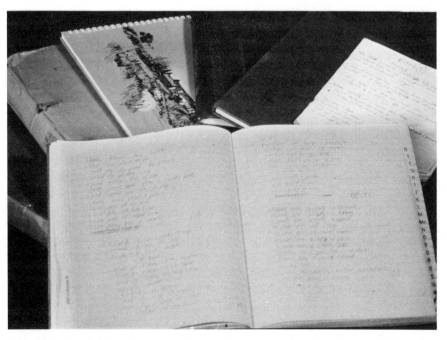

FIG. 8.2A. An example of hypergraphia. A patient brings this large collection of filled notebooks to hospital.

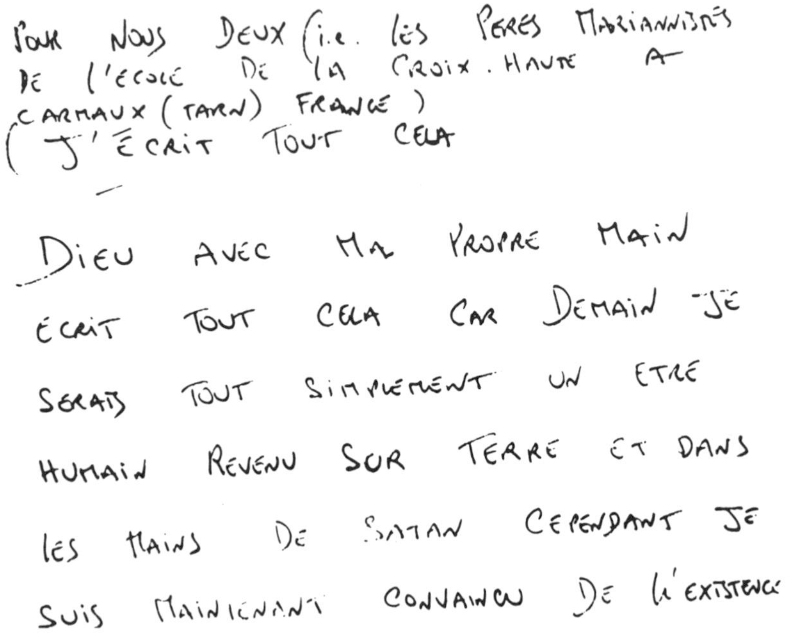

Pour Nous Deux (i.e. les Pères Marianristes
De l'école De la Croix . Haute   a
Carmaux (Tarn) France)
(J'écrit Tout Cela
—

Dieu avec ma propre main

écrit Tout Cela Car Demain Je

Serait Tout Simplement un être

Humain Revenu Sur Terre et dans

les Mains De Satan Cependant Je

Suis Maintenant Convaincu De l'existence

FIG. 8.2B. An example of the religious content from a patient with compulsive hypergraphia. He changes "J'écrit" by crossing it out to "Dieu avec ma propre main ecrit."

striking clinical examples in their reports. They also highlighted stickiness or viscosity, patients showing a striking preoccupation with detail and concerns over moral or ethical issues. Rodin et al. (1984) removed subjects with high and low scores on certain MMPI-derived items from analysis and noted, with cluster analysis, that a cluster corresponding to the epileptic personality was present in association with a temporal lobe seizure disorder in 7% of patients.

Finally, the complexity of these studies has been commented on more recently by Adamec (1989), whose studies have been amongst several identifying mediolimbic seizure disorder as being the form of temporal lobe epilepsy most likely to be associated with psychopathology (see Table 8.2). They gave a modified BFI to 114 patients with epilepsy of varying diagnoses, to 91 psychiatry patients, to 43 patients with chronic illness other than epilepsy, and to 100 normal controls. Three classifications of seizure patients emerged from an item cluster analysis followed by discriminant function analysis; namely, correctly classified seizure patients, those classified as psychiatric patients, and those classified as nonpatients. The 25% classified as psychiatric patients were distinguished from other seizure patients on depression, mood, and metaphysical (religious) clusters and further had 5 of 33 aura experiences more intensely and frequently. These they refer to as limbic auras; namely, formed images, humming or buzzing, irritability, jamais vu, and time changes (see Fig. 8.3).

As shown in Table 8.2, this is one of six studies in which a limbic marker has been used to identify patients with mediolimbic seizures where an association with

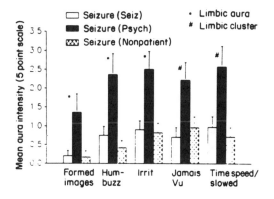

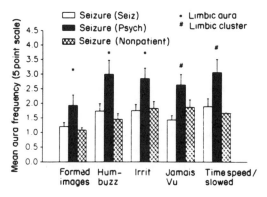

FIG. 8.3. The relationship between limbic auras and psychiatric status in seizure patients and controls is shown in graphs representing mean aura intensity (top) and mean aura frequency (bottom) (Adamec, 1989).

psychopathology has been demonstrated. These include the study of Wieser (1983), using depth electrode recording to verify the site of origin of the seizure in patients with temporal lobe epilepsy. He noted that patients with a medial focus scored higher on a number of the BFI scales when compared with patients with either temporal neocortical involvement or extratemporal foci. Similar links to limbic pathology emerge from the hormonal studies of Dana-Haeri et al. (1984), and the sphenoidal electrode EEG studies of Kristensen and Sindrup (1978) in psychotic patients.

INTERICTAL PSYCHOTIC DISORDERS

Prevalence

Chapter 1 noted the early history of the relationship between epilepsy and psychosis, noting some early studies. Establishing the prevalence of psychosis in patients with epilepsy is hampered by a dearth of investigations, and those that are reported are usually from selected specialist centres. Most early studies do not discriminate between different forms of psychopathology, and the meaning of the term *schizophrenia* has varied over time such that little reliance can be placed upon its use until recent times, when more clearly defined research criteria were introduced to classification.

Echeverria (1873) gives a remarkable figure of 267 psychotic patients amongst 538 epileptics and commented that in no case did he find epilepsy following insanity, the former always occurring first. The literature between 1925 and 1958 was reviewed by Davison and Bagley (1969), and in contrast an average figure from the collected patient sample was 0.7%. These studies do not reveal the prevalence to be significantly greater than that expected of schizophrenia in the general population. However, the authors point out that there are so many uncontrolled variables (for example, age structure, the definition of schizophrenia, and the fact that in many instances the epileptic populations consist of mental hospital inpatients) that little weight could be given to these figures.

Since their review, several other studies are available, again giving remarkably variable figures. The early study of Bartlet (1957) is often quoted in which he examined the case records of patients diagnosed with psychoses following epilepsy at the Bethlem Royal and Maudsley Hospitals from 1949 to 1953. Bartlet included patients who had suffered from delusions for at least a year, and he excluded any patients with schizophrenia complicated by epileptic seizures and epileptic patients with acute psychoses not becoming chronic. He noted twelve psychotic patients, eight diagnosed as schizophrenic, and three with affective psychosis, and gave a prevalence estimate of 0.74%. However, his calculation of the overall number of patients suffering from epilepsy was an estimate based upon correction factors rather than actual cases.

More reliable information can only be derived from community epidemiological surveys where the bias of referral selection is largely removed. Even these studies are open to suspicion, however, since patients who have epilepsy and psychosis may well be away from their community in a special setting, either a psychiatric hospital or a special institution dealing with problems of difficult epilepsy, and these figures are, therefore, an underestimate. Four studies provide information. Pond and Bidwell (1959), in a general practice survey, reported that 7% had been in a mental hospital before or during their survey year and estimated that approximately 10% of the whole group would have a period of inpatient care at some time in their lives. Although a precise figure for psychosis is not derived and no diagnostic categories given, Pond (1974) hints that 7% psychosis is his figure. Gudmundsson (1966) personally examined adult epileptic patients in a comprehensive study in Iceland and was able to compare the prevalence rates of psychiatric disturbances with a general psychiatric survey carried out in Iceland previously by Helgason (1964). He gives a figure of 7.1% as psychotic. Zielinski (1974) provided data on nonselected epileptic patients from Poland. Approximately 3% had psychotic symptoms and 58% showed some "mental abnormality."

In a recent epidemiological survey of general practice patients, Edeh and Toone

(1987) identified 103 patients, of whom only 88 participated in the survey. Of these, 31% had a history of psychiatric referral, and four patients (4.5%) were categorised as currently psychotic.

These studies, reviewed in Table 8.4, particularly the epidemiological surveys, do reveal an increased prevalence of psychosis in epilepsy, although further, more extensive epidemiological investigations using standardized and validated criteria for diagnosis are urgently required. A summary figure of between 4.5% and 7% may be suggested.

As noted, the EEG led to the identification of temporal lobe epilepsy in clinical practice, and the emphasis of the relationship of psychopathology in epilepsy moved from one which suggested no links to the stance adopted by Gibbs (1951), in which psychopathology was associated with temporal lobe abnormalities, particularly anterior temporal discharges. This led to a succession of papers examining this association, information from which is given in Table 8.5. An overrepresentation of patients with temporal lobe abnormalities having severe psychiatric illness was reported by Pond and Bidwell (1959), their temporal lobe epileptics having nearly a 20% hospitalization rate, compared with 7% for the whole group. Likewise, Gudmundsson (1966) reported on overrepresentation of severe psychopathology in those with temporal lobe epilepsy (50%) as opposed to those without temporal lobe epilepsy (24%). With regard specifically to psychosis, Gudmundsson's figures were not all based on personally reviewed cases, and his diagnostic categories are somewhat idiosyncratic. Most of these cases were reported to have grand mal seizures (54%).

Table 8.5 is a summary of the studies that have examined the relationship between different types of epilepsy and psychosis, while Table 8.6 gives the distribution of types of epilepsy in series of psychotic epileptic patients.

TABLE 8.4. *Prevalence of "Insanity" Psychosis or Schizophrenia in Epilepsy*

Author	No. of cases	Prevalence	%
Echeverria (1873)	538	267	50.2
Davison and Bagley (1969) (1925–1958)	8572	59	0.7
Alstrom (1950) (schizophrenia)	897	7	0.8
Gibbs and Gibbs (1952)	2484	219	8.8
Gastaut (1956)	1043	82	7.5
Bartlet (1957) (schizophrenia)	1073	8	0.74
Bruens (1971)	720	17	2.4
Shukla et al. (1979)	132	14	10.6
Onuma et al. (1980)	708	40	5.7
Sengoku (1983)	879	39	4.4
Pond and Bidwell (1959)	—	—	7.0
Gudmundsson (1966)	987	71	7.1
Zielinski (1974)	—	—	3.0
Standage and Fenton (1975)	37	—	8.0
Edeh and Toone (1987)	88	4	4.5
Schmitz and Wolf (1989)	697	28	4.0

TABLE 8.5. *Different Types of Epilepsy and Psychosis; Prevalence of Psychosis in Epilepsy Subgroups.*

Author	TLE		Other focal		Generalised		Mixed	
	N	%	N	%	N	%	N	%
Gibbs and Gibbs, 1952		17		2.0				
Ervin et al., 1955	25/31	81						
Bingley, 1958	5/74	7						
Pond and Bidwell, 1959*		20						7
Stevens, 1966	17/100	17					11/100	11
Small et al., 1966	6/50	12					6/50	12
Small and Small, 1967	0/46	0					1/43	2
Gudmundsson, 1966	5/71	7			38/71	54.0	21/71	30
Curie et al., 1971	12/616	2						
Taylor, 1972†	19/100	19						
Shukla et al., 1979	11/62	18			3/70	4.0		
Jensen and Larsen, 1979b	20/74	27						
Pritchard et al., 1980	6/56	11						
Onuma et al., 1980		9		2.5		3.6		
Ounsted and Lindsay, 1981	9/87	10						
Sherwin, 1981†	7/61	11						
Sherwin et al., 1982†	7/80	9	0/42	0				
Sengoku et al., 1983	21/350	6			14/326	4.0		

*Psychiatric hospitalization
†Temporal lobectomy series

These data should be seen in conjunction with some of the personality studies already discussed above. In particular, the study of Guerrant et al. (1962), who reported that the incidence of psychotic profiles in their temporal lobe group was 23% as opposed to 4% in their medical illness group. Other MMPI studies suggesting elevated psychosis scores in patients with temporal lobe epilepsy or its variants include those of Mignone et al. (1970), Rodin et al. (1976), and Hermann et al. (1982). BFI studies of Bear and Fedio (1977), Hermann and Riel (1981), Nielsen and Kristensen (1981), and Brandt et al. (1985) lead to similar conclusions.

TABLE 8.6. *Psychosis and Epilepsy: TLE and Other Epilepsy Types*

	TLE	Other	Total
Bartlet (1957)	7	1	8
Gastaut et al. (1956)	52	31	83
Guerrant et al. (1962)	7	1	8
Slater and Beard (1963a)	55	14	69
Bruens (1971)	15	1	16
Shukla et al. (1979)	11	3	14
Boudin et al. (1963)	19	8	27
Trimble and Perez (1982)	17	7	24
Parnas et al. (1982)	25	4	29
Garryfallos et al. (1988)	9	0	9
TOTAL:	217	70	287

Studies examining the differences between temporal lobe epilepsy and either other focal epilepsies or generalised seizure disorders are again difficult to interpret, often because of selection bias. The large series reported by Gibbs (Gibbs and Gibbs, 1952) derives largely from nonselective patients, and the incidence of psychosis from their study is shown in Fig. 8.1.

It can be seen that while the incidence of psychosis given here is high in temporal lobe epilepsy (17%), and this is distinct from other focal disorders (2%). The subdivisions suggest that the main psychotic presentations relate to paranoid illness while the incidence of schizophrenia given is low. A problem of interpretation with many earlier studies is the definition of schizophrenia, particularly in North America, where diagnostic criteria for schizophrenia have, until relatively recently, been markedly different from the criteria used by Europeans. Nonetheless, the difference in presentation of psychosis between the temporal lobe group and the other focal group is remarkable.

The studies which fail to distinguish between patients with a temporal lobe focus and others derive largely from one group. Patients were from a medical clinic, meeting strict criteria for either temporal lobe epilepsy or focal or generalised epilepsy. These studies (Small et al., 1966; Small and Small, 1967; Stevens, 1966) compare patients with temporal lobe or psychomotor epilepsy with patients having other focal disorders or generalised seizures of various forms. Little difference is seen between groups although the frequency of schizophrenia in patients with temporal lobe epilepsy is given as up to 17% (a figure consistent with other data already quoted). Stevens (1966) states: "It would be correct to say that nearly two thirds of all the adult epileptics studied who were known to have had psychotic episodes which required hospitalization also had a diagnosis of psychomotor temporal epilepsy" (p. 464). She tempered this with the acknowledgement that in her study the psychomotor-temporal group comprised 54% of the total adult clinic population. In an analysis of individual symptoms, she further noted that "diagnosis of schizophrenia, mood disturbance, anxiety and withdrawal are more common in the psychomotor temporal group". Her data show, in contrast, mental slowing and apathy to be more frequent in a "grand mal diffuse EEG abnormality group" (p. 465).

Stevens interprets this increase in psychosis in her psychomotor group as an age-related phenomena, both epileptic patients and potentially schizophrenic patients increasing the prevalence of mental disorder with increasing age. Why this should relate to schizophrenia but not to mood disturbance, anxiety, mental slowing, and apathy is not quite clear.

Several series show clear differences in the prevalence of psychosis in temporal lobe epilepsy as compared to other epileptic groups, including those of Shukla et al. (1979), Sengoku (1983), Pond and Bidwell (1959), and some studies shown in Table 8.6. Studies of patients with temporal lobe epilepsy only (see Table 8.5) vary from the low frequency of psychosis given by Curie et al. (1971) of 1.8% to the higher figures given by Ounsted and Lindsay (1981) of 10.3%. This latter series was a follow-up study of patients assessed in 1964 of "a large wholly unselective population" of children with epilepsy from which a subgroup of children with temporal lobe epilepsy was drawn. Many variables were coded in 1964, and the children were followed up in 1977. Of the original 100, 87 patients could be followed, and 9 had developed a schizophreniform psychosis. Several additional patients revealed first rank symptoms of Schneider. The figure of 10.3% is, therefore, an underestimate of the number of patients showing psychotic symptoms.

These data complement those of the frequency of psychosis reported in the temporal lobectomy studies, quoted in Chapter 7, which averages 7.4%.

The clear bias towards the temporal lobe group with regard to psychosis is shown in Table 8.6. Although Bartlet (1957) had found only a small number of case histories of epilepsy and psychosis in his series, he commented on the high incidence of EEG and clinical evidence implicating temporal lobe abnormalities, supporting a view which was becoming popular then: that the psychosis was related to temporal lobe dysfunction. As can be seen, all of the series given show temporal lobe epilepsy to be more commonly associated with psychosis, irrespective of the classification of psychosis, an issue to be discussed below.

There are several series of studies of epileptic patients in psychiatric hospitals, and these are given in Table 8.7. Naturally, the frequency is high, the predominant diagnoses being paranoid and schizophrenia-like psychoses. The latter was the specific subject of study of Standage (1973) and formed 40% of the cases of Betts (1981).

Summarising these data, it would seem that there is substantial evidence that psychosis is overrepresented in epilepsy and is further overrepresented in patients with temporal lobe epilepsy compared with other forms of epilepsy. Many of the comparison groups have been patients in whom temporal lobe pathology has not and cannot be excluded. Comparison groups are often patients with generalised seizures, but it is recognised that such patients often show temporal lobe pathology and, indeed, using newer methods of investigation such as video telemetry, it has become appreciated that so-called primary generalised epilepsy often reflects secondarily generalised seizures from a focus. Further, although extratemporal foci have been used in some studies; again, it cannot be assumed that such foci do not generate discharges through the limbic structures and hence cause complex partial seizures.

TABLE 8.7. *Surveys of Epileptic Psychosis in Mental Hospitals*

	Number of cases with epilepsy	Number of psychoses	% psychosis
Liddell (1953)			4.3
Bartlet (1957)	1073	8	0.7
Standage (1973)	53	8	15.1
Betts (1981)	78	47	60.2
Mann and Cree (1976)			5.3
Stevens (1980)	21	2	9.0

Phenomenology

A number of studies in the more recent era emphasise the schizophrenia-like nature of many of the chronic psychoses seen in patients with epilepsy. Earlier examples come from Clark and Lesko (1939), Mulder and Daly (1952), Rodin et al. (1957), and Ervin et al. (1955). The latter group reported a diagnosis of schizophrenia in 81% percent of 42 patients with temporal lobe epilepsy, reaching the conclusion that there was a high correlation between the two. These early authors made the point that the psychiatric symptomatology in the epileptic patients was remarkably similar to schizophrenia noted in nonepileptic patients. The statement of Gibbs (1951) on this point is clear: "The psychiatric symptoms which accompany psychomotor epilepsy are clinically indistinguishable from those encountered in 'purely psychiatric' disorders" (p. 526).

The most important literature stems from the writings of Hill (1953) and Pond (1957). They emphasised the development of chronic paranoid hallucinatory states which were seen especially in temporal lobe epilepsy with complex auras which occurred several years following the onset of seizures, usually in the late teens or twenties. Pond gave an early description of the clinical features:

"They include paranoid ideas which may become systematised, ideas of influence, auditory hallucinations often of a menacing quality, and occasional frank thought disorders with neologisms, condensed words and inconsequential sentences. . . . a religiose colouring of the paranoid ideas is common. The affect tends to remain warm and appropriate, which is sometimes in contrast to 'true schizophrenia,' nor is there typical 'schizophrenic' deterioration to the empty hebephrenic state" (p. 1444).

These features have essentially been confirmed by authors since. The most comprehensive series reported is that of Slater and Beard (1963a). They collected 69 cases from the Maudsley Hospital and the National Hospital, Queen Square, all with clinical diagnoses of epilepsy (supported where possible by EEG evidence) and diagnoses of schizophrenia. They clinically classified the psychoses into three groups: chronic psychosis with recurrent confusional episodes, chronic paranoid states, and hebephrenic states. The most usual onset was insidious, with gradual appearance of delusions, especially in the chronic paranoid subgroup. In 17 cases, the chronic psychosis appeared as a sequel to a series of epileptic confusional episodes; in a further twenty, short-lived psychotic episodes lasting from 11 to 38 days occurred intermittently before the onset of the more chronic disorder. The schizophrenic symptomatology of their subgroups is shown in Table 8.8.

Delusions were shown by all but two of their patients, and in many cases these were religious or mystical (see below). Passivity feelings were prominent, and many patients attributed feelings of special significance to commonplace events. A number of patients claimed special powers; for example, of healing, being able to see through walls or read thoughts, and persecution of an extreme kind was noted in many.

TABLE 8.8. *Schizophrenic Symptomatology, from Self-Description or Observed in Hospital*

	Group A	Group B	Group C	Totals
Delusions in clear consciousness	11	46	10	67
Hallucinations in clear consciousness				
auditory	6	31	9	46
gustatory	—	2	1	3
olfactory	—	4	1	5
somatic	—	5	2	7
visual	3	10	3	16
total patients affected	7	35	10	52
Catatonic disorders of behaviour				
impulsive and bizarre acts	3	6	4	13
loss of mobility and volition	1	12	6	19
manneristic behaviour	3	21	10	34
negativism	1	2	2	5
total patients affected	4	26	10	40
Thought disorder, schizophrenic type	4	16	11	31
Loss of affective responsiveness	1	17	10	28

A = chronic psychoses, B = paranoid states, C = hebephrenic states
(Slater and Beard, 1963a)

Hallucinations, both visual and auditory, were had by 58 patients, the latter being the most common. They were often persecutory voices, but first rank Schneiderian hallucinations were also frequent. Thought disorder was shown by half of the patients, reflected in an inability to handle abstract concepts, a tendency to ramble, and circumstantialities. Also, there was typical schizophrenic thought disorder with thought blocking, neologisms, and evidence of disturbed syntax. Motor disturbances, for example, mannerisms, were frequent, although catatonic phenomena were rare.

Bruens (1971) divided the psychotic syndromes of his patients into four categories. These were paranoid syndromes with delusions (more or less systematised); psychosis with marked mental regression and transient paranoid symptoms; schizophrenia-like psychosis with thought disorders and affective disturbances; and relatively short-lived confusional states. Hallucinations occurred in 78% and were mainly auditory, although visual hallucinations were not uncommon. Delusions were seen in 80% of patients, including delusions of reference, grandeur, and guilt.

The schizophrenia-like presentations in epileptic patients are not confined to Western cultures; they have also been described from countries such as Nigeria (Asuni and Pillutla, 1967), India (Kanaka et al., 1966), and Japan (Sengoku et al., 1983).

Religiosity

The association between epilepsy and religiosity has been commented on in Chapter 1. It has been suggested that a number of well-known mystics and prophets may have suffered epilepsy, but further examples come from more recent times. The case of Swedenborg is an example, as is the case of van Gogh, who not only was an extremely religious man, but may be said to have had other features of the epileptic personality syndrome as described by Geschwind, including hyposexuality and hypergraphia (Appendix). He was also subject to intermittent psychotic bouts.

Examples of patients with epilepsy whose religious feelings appeared to have hypertrophied are discussed by a number of earlier writers, including Echeverria (1873), Clouston (1896), Kraepelin (1923), and Clark and Lesko (1939). The latter authors describe four patients with a chronic schizophrenia-like illness and epilepsy, three of whom had religious delusions or hallucinations. Slater and Beard (1963a) commented that mystical delusions were remarkably common in their series, occurring in 38% of cases. Bruens (1971) noted that "religious contents were fairly common" to the hallucinations of his patients.

There have been few systematic studies of this, but an extensive series was reported by Dewhurst and Beard (1970), who reviewed religious conversions. These had been described in association with epilepsy by Howden (1872, 1873) but, with singular exceptions, cases in the literature were rare. Dewhurst and Beard described six cases, all of whom had temporal lobe epilepsy and were not notably religious prior to their conversion. Out of Slater's 26 cases, only 8 had religious interests prior to the onset of their illness.

Hyperreligiosity was one of the 18 personality traits selected by Bear and Fedio in their studies and, as noted above, results are mixed. It was not associated with a laterality effect or with site of seizure focus in the studies of Nielsen and Kristensen (1981) and other studies did not appear to distinguish temporal lobe epileptics from others where this comparison was made. The exception was the follow-up study of Bear et al. (1982), who noted that religious preoccupations significantly differentiated patients with temporal lobe epilepsy from a mixed psychiatric sample.

Tucker et al. (1987) examined 76 patients with partial complex seizures and gave them the Wiggins Religiosity Scale. The data were compared with those collected from 31 subjects with primary generalised seizures and 27 subjects with pseudoseizures and no epilepsy. No significant differences were noted between groups and neither was there a laterality effect for the temporal lobe epilepsy sample. Willmore et al. (1980) compared 20 patients with temporal lobe epilepsy to 14 with generalised epilepsy on a specially designed 154-item questionnaire assessing various aspects of religiosity, and differences were noted between the groups on only 17 items, the generalised epilepsy groups scoring in the more religious direction.

The negative results from questionnaire studies, which stand in contrast to the longstanding clinical observations, require further investigation and explanation. It is most likely that, as with hypergraphia, religiosity in patients with epilepsy is either culturally appropriate and has therefore been of less clinical interest; or pathological, in which case it is an all-or-none phenomenon and is seen in only a minority of patients. It would not, therefore, necessarily emerge as a prominent factor in questionnaire studies unless a sufficiently large number of patients was evaluated.

Types of Psychosis and Types of Seizures

It is the criticism of much of the work in the area of epilepsy and psychosis that the latter term has been used without definition, and little attempt has been made to specify the precise phenomenology of patients examined. The importance of such precision has been emphasised by studies that have used standardized and validated methods of quantifying psychopathology in the psychoses. In the first report of this kind, Perez and Trimble (1980) described the mental state of patients with epilepsy and psychosis, prospectively referred, with psychoses lasting longer than a month in a setting of clear consciousness. They were evaluated using the PSE (Wing et al., 1974). This is a semistandardised technique which allows for categorisation of patients' symptoms by use of the Catego computer programme, and the authors were able to compare the PSE syndrome profile for the epileptic sample with a control nonepileptic schizophrenic group. They found that 50% of the patients with epilepsy and psychosis were categorised as having schizophrenic psychosis, 92% having a profile of nuclear schizophrenia based on the first rank symptoms of Schneider (Table 8.9).

The syndrome profile of the patients with schizophrenia and epilepsy compared with those with schizophrenia showed few significant differences, emphasising the similarities of the clinical presentation of these two disorders. In this sample, 17 patients had complex partial seizures and a history of an EEG abnormality compatible with a diagnosis of temporal lobe epilepsy. In seven the seizure type was generalised, and a diagnosis of primary or secondary generalised epilepsy was made. When the PSE subclass diagnosis of the epileptic psychotic patients were examined by epilepsy diagnosis, eleven of the temporal lobe group were categorised as having nuclear schizophrenia (NS), and six had other forms of psychoses. None of the generalised group had a diagnosis of NS. As can be seen in Table 8.10, non-schizophrenia-like psychoses were also recorded, in particular, paranoid and affective psychoses.

TABLE 8.9. *Catego Subclasses and Classes—Diagnostic Comparison Between Epileptic Psychotic and Schizophrenic Patients*

Subclass diagnoses	Epileptics (n = 24)	Schizophrenics (n = 11)
Nuclear schizophrenia	11	9
Schizophrenia without first rank symptoms	1	—
Residual schizophrenia/mania	1	—
Manic psychosis	3	—
Psychotic depression	3	1
Paranoid psychosis/retarded depression	3	—
Paranoid psychosis/affective psychosis	1	—
Paranoid psychosis	1	1
Total	24	11

(Trimble and Perez, 1982)

TABLE 8.10. Catego Subclasses and Classes—Diagnostic Comparison Between Patients with Temporal Lobe and Generalised Epilepsy

Catego subclasses	TLE (n = 18)	GEN (n = 7)
Nuclear schizophrenia	11	—
Schizophrenia without first rank symptoms	—	1
Residual schizophrenia/mania	—	1
Manic psychosis	1	2
Psychotic depression	1	2
Paranoid psychosis/retarded depression	3	—
Paranoid psychosis/affective psychosis	1	—
Paranoid psychosis	1	1

(Trimble and Perez, 1982)
(TLE) temporal lobe epilepsy, (GEN) generalised epilepsy

In Fig. 8.4, the PSE syndrome profile of 11 patients with temporal lobe epilepsy and NS is compared with that of 9 nonepileptic schizophrenic controls, also rated as NS. The profiles are very similar, two exceptions being delusions of grandeur and visual hallucinations, both of which were significantly more common in the non-epileptic group.

Thirteen of the total sample of patients with epilepsy and psychosis received a diagnosis other than nuclear schizophrenia; six came from the temporal lobe group.

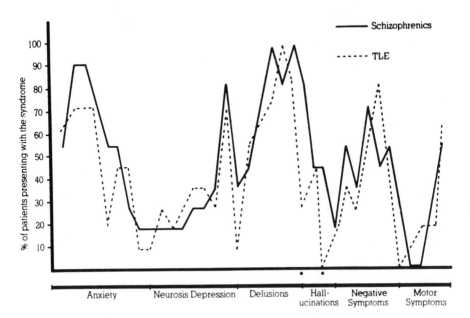

FIG. 8.4. The PSE syndromes of patients with schizophrenia and no epilepsy and those with a schizophrenia-like psychosis and temporal lobe epilepsy. Note the close similarity of the profiles.

Affective disorders were noted. All the temporal lobe patients had either a primary or a combined disturbance of affect, and in four out of six the combination was with a paranoid psychosis. Generalised epilepsy was less clearly related to a disorder of affect, and paranoid psychoses were rare (one out of seven). Examination of syndrome profiles of the two subgroups revealed the temporal lobe group to show more delusions of persecution and of reference and more special features of depression than the generalised group, the latter showing more tension, sexual fantasies, overactivity, depersonalization, and hypomania.

Toone et al. (1982 a) used the Syndrome Check List derived from the PSE in a retrospective study of 69 patients with a combined diagnosis of epilepsy and psychosis, and compared the profiles with 13 patients with functional psychosis. When patients in the schizophrenia-like index group were examined, they displayed less catatonia but had more delusions of persecution and of reference than controls.

These data suggest that in a group of patients with psychosis and epilepsy a significant number have a schizophrenia-like presentation with many features similar to nuclear schizophrenia in the absence of epilepsy. Exceptions to this include the motor symptoms and preservation of affect, noted by Slater and Beard (1963a,b) and discussed further below. There are also suggestions that patients with temporal lobe epilepsy have a different profile of psychosis than patients with generalised seizure disorders. Trimble and colleagues emphasised the presentation of NS in association with temporal lobe pathology. Patients with psychoses and generalised epilepsies have a variety of psychopathological presentations, which include schizophrenia without first rank symptoms and manic and depressive psychoses.

These data confirm a direct link between certain types of epilepsy and certain patterns of clinical presentation hinted at in the early reports of Pond (1957), which can also be noted in some other studies (Table 8.11). Stevens (1966) drew attention to the diagnosis of schizophrenia in association with psychomotor temporal lobe epilepsy, in contrast to mental slowing and apathy which were more frequent with grand mal, diffuse EEG abnormality patients. Bruens (1971) noted that the majority of his patients with temporal lobe epilepsy showed psychoses of a paranoid or regressive nature, primarily generalised epilepsy being associated more with confu-

TABLE 8.11. *Schizophrenic, Paranoid, Confusional, and Dysphoric Psychoses in Generalised and Temporal Lobe Epilepsy*

Author	TLE		GEN	
	S	C	S	C
Dongier (1959, 1960)	49	20	12	64
Shukla et al. (1979)	92	18	43	57
Dorr-Zegers and Rauh (1980)	83	17	23	77
Bruens (1980)	58	42	22	77
Perez and Trimble (1980)	69	31	28	72
%	70.2	25.6	25.6	70.0

(S) schizophrenic and paranoid psychoses, (C) confusional and dysphoric psychoses, (TLE) temporal lobe epilepsy, (GEN) generalised epilepsy.

sional psychosis. Slater and Beard (1963a) noted that the majority of their group with centrencephalic epilepsy showed hebephrenic features (five out of seven).

A comprehensive evaluation of the EEG manifestations of psychotic episodes occurring interictally was presented by Dongier (1959, 1960). The clinical presentations associated with 536 psychotic episodes occurring in 516 epileptic patients interictally were documented following considerable briefing in order to attempt to verify the various concepts and terminologies employed by different investigators. Forty-four percent of psychotic episodes were associated with generalised discharges, 16% with focal discharges, the majority of those (11.6%) being temporal. With regard to the normalisation story (see Chapter 5), disappearance of the EEG abnormalities during the psychotic episode was seen in 24% of cases, mainly of a focal or bisynchronous discharge. Over half of the psychotic episodes were associated with alteration of the state of consciousness and of the remainder, 30% showed predominantly affective disorders, the rest showing schizophrenia-like presentations or pure hallucinosis. Confusional symptoms were more frequent in patients with centrencephalic seizures, these presentations often being associated with diffuse delta waves or more or less continuous bisynchronous spike-and-wave discharges on the EEG. Affective disorders were not closely associated with epilepsy type, but focal epilepsies tended to show more depression (45% of temporal lobe epilepsy cases compared with 24% of centrencephalics). Delusions were more frequent among focal epilepsies, especially where a preexisting focal discharge disappeared. In this group, the duration of the psychosis was often several days or weeks, in contrast to the briefer psychotic episodes often seen with more generalised EEG disturbances. Finally, the schizophrenia-like presentations were more often associated with temporal lobe epilepsy (20% compared with 12% in centrencephalic cases). In summary, Dongier's data show differences in the presentation of psychosis between psychomotor epilepsy and generalised epilepsy, the former presenting more affective disorders and schizophrenia-like or paranoid presentations.

Similar data, emphasising the association between focal seizures, especially with complex symptomatology and prolonged psychosis with schizophrenia-like symptoms, in contrast to briefer episodes of dysphoric nonparanoid psychoses often associated with confusion, derives from the figures of Dorr-Zegers and Rauh (1980) (83% schizophrenia-like illnesses in temporal lobe epilepsy against 23% in generalised disorders), in a retrospective series collected over twenty years from Heidelberg. Bruens (1980) provided information on 57 epileptic patients suffering from psychosis from the Hans Berger clinic and gives equivalent figures of 58% and 22%. As can be seen from Table 8.11, there is a considerable conformity of data on this point.

Affective States

As noted above, several authors comment on affective disorders in association with psychosis of epilepsy, although discussion of affective psychosis per se is rare.

It has been recognised for many years that epileptic patients may suffer from depressive symptoms (Griesinger, 1857), and in the early descriptions of ictally related changes of the mental state, excitement, manic presentation, and overactivity were notable (Morel, 1860). Ictally related affective disorders, particularly mania, have been discussed in Chapter 6, but interictal affective psychoses, in particular, classical manic or bipolar pictures are considered rare. Admittedly, in many early studies, operational criteria were not used to distinguish different forms of psychoses, and paranoid affective states may have been common. The series that report affective psychoses are singularly few. Gibbs and Gibbs (1952) noted 4.2% of 678 cases of psychomotor epilepsy to have manic-depressive illness or depression, and 2.8% had suicidal tendencies.

Curie et al. (1971) noted only 4 of 666 cases to have a severe depressive illness, a remarkably low figure.

Bartlet reported 1 depressive and 2 manic psychoses in his series of 11; Bruens (1980) had 3 depressive psychoses out of 57 (1 generalised epilepsy), while Dorr-Zegers and Rauh (1980) had 3 cases: 2 bipolar illnesses, both with focal seizures. Perez and Trimble (1980) noted 8 cases out of 23, equally divided between temporal lobe and generalised seizure types.

Toone and colleagues (1982), using the SCL, noted 16 cases (23%) which, when compared to nonepileptic patients with similar psychopathology, were more likely to be male and to have multiple, recurrent episodes.

Dongier (1959, 1960) reported 47 cases of depressive episodes and 20 of manic episodes, the distribution of centrencephalic and temporal forms of epilepsy being similar for the two groups. As noted, patients who showed normalisation, particularly of a preexisting focus, frequently presented with affective disturbances as part of their psychotic episodes. However, it is not clear that any of her examples represented more classical manic-depressive psychoses.

Betts (1974) reported endogenous depression to be the principal psychiatric diagnosis of 17% of 72 patients admitted to mental hospital, although it is not clear how many of these patients were psychotic.

The highest frequency of affective psychosis was reported by Fenton (1978), who noted 6 patients with an affective psychosis of a total of 14 psychotic patients in a sample of 80 consecutive admissions of epileptic patients to the Maudsley Hospital. Five more had a schizoaffective disorder, thus making 11 of 14 with an affective or schizoaffective psychosis (78%).

Robertson et al. (1987) carried out a comprehensive survey of the phenomenology of interictal depressive states in 66 consecutively referred cases. Thirteen were psychotic (19.6%), although bipolar presentations were rare.

A number of authors have commented on the frequency of suicide in epilepsy (Marchand and Ajuriaguerra, 1948; Barraclough, 1981) which seems especially high for patients with temporal lobe epilepsy. However, it cannot be assumed that such patients are necessarily psychotic.

The most interesting study of affective psychoses in epilepsy is that of Flor-Henry (1969) referred to in Chapter 9. All his cases had temporal lobe epilepsy, and manic-depressive states were characterised by euphoric or depressive alterations of mood, exhibiting periodicity but leaving the personality intact between phases. Of 50 cases, 11 were schizoaffective and 9 manic-depressive (40%).

Summarizing these data, it is clear that affective psychoses have been much less the subject of study than the schizophrenia-like illnesses and, with the singular exception of Flor-Henry's highly selected series of patients with temporal lobe epilepsy, the majority report manic illness to be infrequent and classical bipolar affective disorders to be rare. Depressive psychoses are more common, figures varying from the 2% reported by Bruens to the 78% reported by Fenton.

What is clear is that affective symptoms are often intermixed with psychotic symptoms in the classical schizophrenia-like psychoses. This emerged from the extensive study of Slater and Beard (1963a) who noted affective disturbance shown by all of their patients, usually in the form of periodic moods of depression or irritability. The mood swings were described as short lived and severe, and in nearly 50% of patients one or more attempts of suicide were made during such states. Ecstasy was reported by 17% of the patients, most typically as a semimystical experience. Flatness of affect was reported in 40%, but generally, particularly in relationship to classical schizophrenia, the patients retained affective warmth, and this was one of the characteristic distinguishing features between the schizophrenia-like psychoses of epilepsy and process schizophrenia.

9

Interictal Psychoses
Risk Factors

RISK FACTORS

A number of risk factors which may be associated with the development of psychosis and epilepsy are listed in Table 9.1. These are individually discussed.

Age of Onset of Seizures and Relationship to Age of Onset of Psychosis

The significance of age of onset of seizures for the development of psychopathology was noted in the MMPI study of Hermann et al. (1980) where a group of patients with temporal lobe epilepsy, in contrast to those with other forms of epilepsy, were shown to have higher elevations of psychotic subscales with an adolescent onset of seizures (aged 13 to 18). The age of onset of seizures, in samples from which it can be determined, is shown in Table 9.2. It is clear that the mean age of onset is usually in early adolescence. However, controlled series do not reveal differences between psychotic and nonpsychotic groups. For example, Flor-Henry (1969) gives figures of 13 years for his psychotic sample and 18 for a control group. The figures of Kristensen and Sindrup (1978a) are 10 and 12 years, respectively, and Sengoku et al. (1983) give 14.2 and 14.9 years. Ounsted and Lindsay were unable to relate age of onset to the later development of a schizophrenia-like illness.

Far more attention has been given to the interval between the age of onset epilepsy and the age of the onset of psychosis. This was first discussed in detail by Beard (1963). In Slater's series, the interval was significantly less for those patients developing hebephrenic states. The mean interval for the entire series was 14 years, and they noted a correlation coefficient of 0.48 between the ages of onsets of epilepsy and psychosis. They gave this as one reason for suggesting an aetiological relationship between epileptic seizures and psychosis.

As shown in Table 9.2, with the exception of the Scandinavian series, there is a remarkable homogeneity of the interval, being in the region of 11 to 15 years. Perez

TABLE 9.1. *Risk Factors Associated with Psychosis of Epilepsy*

Age of onset:	Early adolescence
Interval:	Onset of seizures to onset of psychosis: ~14 years
Sex:	Bias to females
Seizure type:	Complex partial: automatisms
Seizure frequency:	Diminished, especially temporal lobe
Seizure focus:	Temporal, especially left-sided
Neurological findings:	Sinistrality
	Pathology: gangliogliomas, hamartomas
EEG:	Forced normalization in a subgroup
	Mediobasal focus

and Trimble (1980) have made the point that subcategories of psychoses differ and noted the significantly shorter interval in patients with nuclear syndromes.

This mean interval has come in for considerable discussion. Slater's data was criticised because no case occurred in which the onset of psychosis was before the onset of the epilepsy (Slater and Moran, 1969). The authors reexamined their data, taking these facts into account, and they tested statistically whether epilepsy had an influence on the distribution of the age of first admission for the schizophrenia-like illness. They noted that for both males and females the psychosis occurred earlier than would be expected, but this was only significant for females.

TABLE 9.2. *Age of Onset of Epilepsy and Interval to Onset of Psychosis*

Author	Age at seizure onset	Interval (years)
Gastaut (1956)	20	11
Slater and Beard (1963a)	15	14
Jus (1966)		13
Flor-Henry (1969)	13[a]	14
Davison and Bagley (1969)	15	15
Bruens (1971)	13	12
Standage (1973)		19
Kristensen and Sindrup (1978a,b)	10[b]	21
Jensen and Larsen (1979b)	14	14
Dorr-Zegers and Rauh (1980)		15
Trimble and Perez (1980)	11[c]	16[d]
Parnas et al. (1982)		22
Sengoku et al. (1983)	14[e]	14
Schmitz and Wolf (1989)		13
	MEAN	15

[a]Controls, 18
[b]Controls, 12
[c]Nuclear schizophrenia, 11, nonnuclear schizophrenia, 9
[d]Nuclear schizophrenia, 16, nonnuclear schizophrenia, 27
[e]Controls, 14

Male/female differences in relationship to age of onset were further examined by Taylor (1971). Using the data provided by Slater and Beard (1963a), he pointed out there was a large excess of females who had both onset of epilepsy and psychosis before they were 20 years old. In general, those patients who developed psychosis had onset of epilepsy around puberty, which was significantly later than patients in a control group who had been referred for temporal lobectomy and did not have psychosis. This led Taylor to suggest that a different aetiology was related to the seizure disorder in the two groups, and that cerebral maturation differed between the sexes. He summarized this by suggesting that females have a higher risk for the development of psychosis, but that this risk is passed by the age of 25 years.

Sex

The various series reported show a relatively even distribution of gender, some with more males (Slater and Beard, 1963a), others with more females (Kristensen and Sindrup, 1978a). However, Taylor (1971) noted that the sex ratio in epilepsy generally shows a bias towards males, giving figures of 135 males to 100 females from Department of Health and Social Security data. His own analysis of Slater's cases suggests an increased risk in females, and he has provided further confirmation from the temporal lobectomy cases of Falconer (Taylor, 1975). Of 88 cases, psychosis was more common in females (24%) than in males (9%).

Seizure Variables

The association between temporal lobe epilepsy and psychosis has already been emphasized, and the specific relationship between certain forms of psychosis, particularly presenting with paranoid or nuclear schizophrenia-like symptoms and temporal lobe lesions, has been suggested. It is not surprising, therefore, that most studies report that patients with psychoses have complex partial seizures, sometimes associated with secondary generalization. In Slater's series these were more common in those with chronic psychoses of a paranoid or recurrent nature, as opposed to the hebephrenic group.

There are two controlled series available. That of Flor-Henry (1969) reported more infrequent psychomotor attacks in his psychotic sample. Kristensen and Sindrup (1978a,b) noted a higher frequency of automatisms or automatisms with epigastric or déjà vu auras in their psychotic group. There was no difference in the incidence of generalised seizures.

Schmitz and Wolf (1989), in a survey of 28 psychotic patients who attended a neurological outpatient clinic, noted that psychoses were significantly more frequent in patients with complex as opposed to simple partial seizures.

The relationship between seizure frequency and psychosis has been examined in a different fashion by several authors, noting the relationship of the onset of the psychosis to the seizures themselves. No clear relationship was observed by Hill et al.

(1957), Glaser (1964), or Small et al. (1966). In contrast, Stevens noted 10 out of 13 psychomotor temporal lobe epileptic patients with psychosis who decompensated during a remission for seizures, often brought about by a change of seizure therapy. In contrast, four out of five grand mal patients appeared to have an exacerbation of their psychosis in association with increased seizures and worsening of the EEG.

Bruens (1971) had 5 out of 19 patients (26%) who showed diminished epileptic activity during the psychosis, 4 of these having evidence of a temporal lobe focus. In Slater's series, only grand mal attacks were taken into account, and no clear relationship emerged. Flor-Henry (1969) suggested that this negative result was because other forms of seizures were ignored, since his own study demonstrated that psychotic patients exhibited fewer seizures, in particular, fewer psychomotor and what he referred to as minor temporal seizures, when compared to a control group. When seizure frequency and type of psychosis were examined, he noted that affective psychoses were correlated with major convulsive epilepsy infrequently manifested.

Kristensen and Sindrup (1978a,b) did not note differences with regard to generalised seizures when psychotics were compared with controls, but did notice a diminished seizure frequency for complex partial seizures.

While acknowledging that assessment of seizure frequency is difficult, particularly retrospectively, as is the case in the studies quoted, the controlled studies both suggest a diminished frequency of psychomotor temporal lobe seizures in patients developing psychosis; there are several reports of individual patients who have some antithetical relationship between seizures and psychosis which would seem to be of importance. These data suggest that there is a subgroup of patients where such a relationship does hold. This may be viewed as a form of antagonism between seizures and psychosis, a variant of the phenomena described by Landolt, as in some cases the EEG is shown to normalise (see below).

Several authors have noted the association between psychosis and more than one seizure type (e.g., Bruens, 1971; Parnas et al., 1982; Schmitz and Wolf, 1989), usually with secondary generalisation from focal seizures.

EEG Studies

The series reported by Dongier (1959, 1960) has already been referred to above. Clear evidence of forced normalisation was shown in 24% of cases, especially in relationship to focal temporal discharges. Other findings can be briefly summarized. Patients showing more or less continuous bisynchronous spike-and-wave discharges were generally confused, as were those showing diffuse slow waves. Patients whose EEG was the same as that taken before the psychotic episode commonly presented with mood swings and depression, while those whose discharges disappeared during the episodes were more significantly reported to show paranoid behaviour.

Bruens (1971) noted forced normalization in five cases, while the EEG investigations of Slater's series (Beard, 1963) revealed the preponderance of temporal lobe abnormalities, as already discussed. Kristensen and Sindrup (1978b) compared the EEG findings of 96 patients with partial epileptic seizures and complex automatisms with psychosis to findings of a control group with epilepsy and no psychosis. There was no difference between the groups with regard to the frequency of patients with focal spike activity during either the waking or sleeping EEG, but highly significant differences were noted with regard to sphenoidal recordings. Thus, sphenoidal spikes were recorded in 82% of psychotics as opposed to 41% of controls. No significant difference was noted in the location of temporal lobe spikes, in relationship to whether they were anterior, medial or posterior temporal; but psychotic patients exhibited a significantly higher number of independent spikes, and their background activity more frequently showed an admixture of diffuse slow-wave activity. The mediobasal temporal lobe abnormalities as located with sphenoidal electrodes in psychotic patients represent another study showing links between medial-limbic disturbances and psychosis (see Table 8.2).

Ramani and Gumnit (1982) have reported the only study of intensive monitoring of interictal psychoses of epilepsy. In reality, their cases were largely ictally related phenomena in the sense that they had been admitted to hospital for control of intractable seizures, and they experienced a psychotic episode while in hospital, the duration of which varied from 1 to 3 weeks. It is not clarified whether the episode recorded was of the same character as the chronic psychosis from which a number suffered, the duration of the psychotic illness varying from 1 to 30 years. Nine had a schizophrenia-like psychosis, the majority having paranoid presentations. Six patients had interictal temporal lobe spikes, two had primary generalised epilepsy, and two patients had generalised bursts of synchronous frontocentrally predominant slow spike-and-polyspike-wave discharges. One patient showed a striking reduction of seizures and EEG normalization. No unequivocal changes in the EEGs were recorded in the other patients. Two patients, in addition to the one showing normalization, showed alternating psychoses, the control of their seizures being related to the emergence of the psychosis.

Neurological Features

Findings at neurological examination or following psychometric testing are omitted from many series. Jensen and Larsen (1979b) comment that their psychotic patients "appeared to be intellectually brighter" than nonpsychotics, while the average IQ of the sample of Toone et al. (1982a) was 96.

Perez and Trimble (1980) noted a difference in the intellectual performance of their subgroups, depending on the categorization of the psychosis. In particular, those with nuclear schizophrenia were shown to have an IQ significantly superior to those patients with other forms of psychosis, the patients with nuclear schizophrenia coming from a large group that had temporal lobe epilepsy. Beard (1963) reported lack of spontaneity, slowness, and retardation in 34 cases, impaired memory in 29 cases, and viscosity in 22. They said only 13 of their patients (19%) were free of any indication of organic personality change. However, they acknowledged that these findings were subjective.

Flor-Henry (1969) noted more abnormal neurological examinations and brain damage in the schizophrenic patients as opposed to manic depressive epileptic patients, the latter having higher IQ (92 and 105, respectively). Kristensen and Sindrup (1978a) noted that the clinical neurological examination showed positive signs of organic damage in only a small proportion of their patients, but this was significantly greater in the psychotic sample compared with controls (13% and 5%, respectively). In addition, they reported that their psychotic patients had a significant increase in left-handers or ambidextrals (16 out of 92) compared with controls (5 out of 95). Such an increase in sinistrality had been earlier commented on by Taylor (1975), in whose series 7 out of 13 psychotic patients were left-handed compared to 11 out of 75 nonpsychotic patients. Further, more patients with an alien tissue lesion were left-handed. When considering the latter group only, two three-way interactions were noted by Taylor between sex, psychosis, and handedness; and sex, psychosis, and side of operation. These highlighted the excess of psychotic females, the absence of psychosis in right-handed males, and the excess of left-sided surgical operations. Taylor felt that left-handedness represented "unusual organization of cerebral function," and stressed that it did not necessarily mean a shift of dominance to the alternative hemisphere.

Radiological Studies

Air encephalography (PEG) was carried out in 56 of 69 cases of Slater and Beard (1963a), and was reported normal in 17. The main abnormality was atrophy (36) in 19 cases there being dilatation of one or both temporal horns, either as part of generalised ventricular dilatation or by itself. Temporal horn abnormalities were exclusively defined in the groups with chronic psychoses and recurrent confusional episodes or the chronic paranoid states and not noted in the hebephrenics. Sherwin (1977) noted abnormal PEG in 18 of 23 patients with psychosis and epilepsy; in 14 there was temporal horn dilatation. Flor-Henry (1969) reported that 52% of his schizophrenia-like psychoses had air encephalographic abnormalities, but this was not significantly different from 58% found in nonpsychotic controls. Kristensen and Sindrup (1978a) also failed to note differences between their psychotics and controls.

Computerized tomography studies have been carried out by Trimble and colleagues (Perez et al., 1985) and Toone et al. (1982b). The former group used visual inspection and linear measurements to compare patients with epilepsy and nuclear schizophrenia (as rated on the PSE) with epileptic nonnuclear schizophrenia and a group of nonepileptic schizophrenic patients. The psychotic groups generally showed higher values for measurements of the bilateral septum caudate distance, the third ventricular size, cistern-brainstem ratio, and the fourth ventricular ratio. The only significant difference between the epileptic samples was that the nonnuclear schizophrenic group showed a smaller cella media size. Laterality differences were examined, and none were noted in patients with a Catego diagnosis of nuclear schizophrenia.

Toone et al. (1982b) compared 57 patients with epilepsy and psychosis with 78 controls with a diagnosis of epilepsy and a psychiatric illness other than psychosis. Abnormalities were reported in 44% of the index and 50% of the control subjects. No differences were noted when diagnostic subgroups were examined comparing schizophrenic, affective, and paranoid patients. Laterality differences were noted, which are discussed further below.

There is one study of CT attenuation densities of patients with epilepsy and psychiatric disorder in which 12 patients with a schizophrenia-like psychosis of epilepsy were evaluated (White et al., unpublished manuscript). No significant relationships were found between regional CT and any clinical parameter, although the frontal densities and left temporal densities were nonsignificantly lower in the schizophrenia-like psychoses compared with nonpsychotic patients.

Conlon and Trimble (1990) examined T1 values on MRI in a group of patients with epileptic psychosis and compared these data to epileptic patients with no history of psychiatric illness. No differences were noted between the two groups, either on visual inspection of the scans or on the quantitative analysis. However, within the psychotic patients, those who had hallucinations of a first rank nature had significantly higher T1 values in the left temporal white matter, compared with those who did not have hallucinations.

Trimble and colleagues also carried out an interictal study of epilepsy which included an examination of psychotic patients using positron emission tomography (PET) (Gallhofer et al., 1985). Using Oxygen 15, regions of interest were used to calculate absolute quantitive values for regional cerebral blood flow (rCBF), regional oxygen extraction ratio (rOER) and regional metabolic rate for oxygen (rCMRO$_2$). Six psychotic patients, all with complex partial seizures and secondary generalization, and five out of six presenting with first rank symptoms of Schneider, were compared with five age-matched, nonpsychotic epileptic patients and age-matched, nonepileptic volunteer controls. The psychotic patients were free from antipsychotic drugs for varying intervals from 9 days in one patient to two patients who had never received such treatment. Figure 9.1 is taken from the Trimble study. Psychotic patients had lower rCMRO$_2$, higher rCBF, and lower rOER in the majority of regions of interest examined, compared with nonpsychotic epileptics. Left- and right-sided values were compared, and the psychotic group had significantly lower values for rCBF and rCMRO$_2$ on the left side across the entire temporal cortex, opposite to the trend seen for nonpsychotic patients, with the exception of the anterior temporal rCMRO$_2$.

In other studies (Bernardi et al., 1984), this group had shown that patients with temporal lobe epilepsy show hypometabolic zones in the temporal cortex corresponding to the focus on their EEGs. The hypometabolism was extensive in the

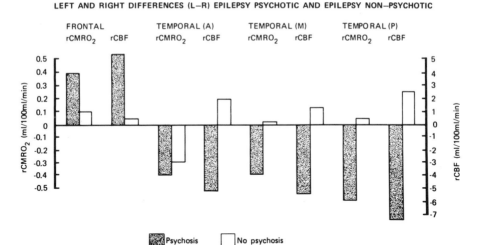

FIG. 9.1. Patients with psychosis and epilepsy have lower values for rCMRO$_2$ and rCBF in the left temporal regions compared with controls. Values shown are L = R differences. Study using PET and Oxygen = 15.

sense of affecting frontal areas and basal ganglia on the side of the lesion. These metabolic changes are more extensive than the subtle areas of more localised structural change detected with, for example, MRI (Conlon and Trimble, 1990).

These radiological studies suggest that patients with epilepsy and psychosis probably do not differ from controls in relationship to the gross amount of ventricular dilatation seen, but studies using CT, MRI, and PET do suggest differences between psychotic patients and controls, particularly with regard to the involvement of the left hemisphere, possibly in association with certain psychotic symptoms such as hallucinations. This issue of laterality is discussed further below. Changes in function as revealed through PET seem greater than changes of structure.

Family History

A number of authors have commented on the family history of psychosis or epilepsy in their samples, the most intensive investigation being that of Slater and Glithero (1963). In this study, accessible relatives were interviewed and emphasis was not placed, therefore, only on hospital records or the patient's own knowledge. Third-party information was available on 88% of patients. Amongst the relatives were noted eight epileptics, two schizophrenics, and twelve patients with psychopathic personalities. By using mathematical calculations of the expected risk, they concluded that the incidence of schizophrenia amongst the relatives was that expected from a sample of the general population. They noted that this was remarkably different from the expectation, had their subjects been schizophrenics where heritability has been established. Similarly, no excess of schizophrenia was found in relatives in the studies of Flor-Henry (1969) or Perez et al. (1985). Kristensen and Sindrup (1978a) noted a positive family history of epilepsy to be more frequent in their control patients.

The only study to suggest a significant hereditary component to the psychopathology of epilepsy was that of Jensen and Larsen (1979b). They noted major psychiatric disorders in 65% of the relatives of their psychotic patients, compared with 39% in relatives of nonpsychotics. These were patients being evaluated for temporal lobectomy. The study of Slater and colleagues is the only one which evaluated genetic aspects comprehensively; it was carried out by authors well-versed in genetic methodology.

Metabolic Aspects

The relationship of abnormal folate metabolism to psychiatric disorders in general, and to those of epilepsy in particular, has been of interest since the early publications of Reynolds (1967). He postulated that a deficiency of folate, brought about by anticonvulsant treatment, may lead to psychopathology, particularly dementia and schizophrenia-like illnesses in epilepsy. He described a series of cases involving schizophrenia-like psychoses with anticonvulsant-drug-induced megaloblastic anaemia or nonanaemic folate deficiency. In one case a clear inverse relationship between seizures and psychosis was noted, leading Reynolds to suggest a significant role of folate deficiency, folate being a significant CNS methyl donor, in the development of psychosis.

Bruens (1971) noted diminished folate levels in five cases where it was measured, while Ramani and Gumnit (1982) noted that most of their patients had low serum folate levels, but these were no different from nonpsychotic epileptic patients in their unit.

The role of folate is inextricably bound with that of anticonvulsants, and several authors have examined prescriptions in relationship to psychosis. The results do not suggest an association between the interictal psychoses and prescribed drugs (Slater and Beard, 1963a,b; Flor-Henry, 1969; Bruens, 1971; Perez et al., 1985). It is, however, recognised that individual patients may develop a psychosis associated with anticonvulsant drugs, and such literature is noted in Chapter 10. Further, intoxication occasionally produces an organic psychosyndrome, but this is different from the kind of psychoses being considered here.

There is one CSF report, that of Peters (1979), who compared CSF monoamine metabolites in a group of psychotic and nonpsychotic patients with temporal lobe epilepsy using the probenecid technique. The psychosis was determined by the use of the MMPI, and CSF homovanillic acid (HVA) was found to be lower in the psychotic sample. This intriguing finding requires replication, but is consistent with abnormalities of dopamine metabolism in association with psychosis, especially upregulation of postsynaptic receptors leading to decreased synaptic dopamine release and breakdown.

Laterality

Flor-Henry (1969) was the first to discuss the issue of laterality in relationship to psychosis and epilepsy. In his study, 18% of all cases of psychosis lateralised to the right hemisphere, in contrast to 50% of the controls. Further, when bilateral cases were taken into account, he found that with respect to psychosis, bilateral and unilateral left foci were equivalent. When left-sided and bilateral foci were compared to right-sided lesions, a highly significant excess of psychotics was noted in the former. With regard to type of psychosis, Flor-Henry reported the highest incidence of right-sided unilateral (nondominant) foci in manic depressives, while in schizophrenic patients, the dominant lobe was mainly involved. This issue has been taken up by a number of other authors, the combined data from surveys where it is possible to establish the laterality of the focus being shown in Table 9.3.

Slater and Beard (1963a,b) looked for a laterality effect but did not find it. Flor-Henry suggested that if laterality effects are important, they may have been obscured by the high proportion of bilateral foci. In general, with the exception of the Scandinavian findings (Kristensen and Sindrup, 1978a,b), there is a clear bias towards a left-sided abnormality, coming from different samples collected in different ways. The follow-up study of Ounsted and Lindsay (1981) required that the laterality of the focus was established 13 years prior to the follow-up, minimising any bias that could have crept in. Nine of their patients had developed schizophrenia-

TABLE 9.3. *Laterality and Epileptic Psychosis*

Author	Left	Right	Bilateral	Total
Slater and Beard (1963a,b)	16	12	20	48
Flor-Henry (1969)	19	9	22	50
Taylor (1975)	9	4	0	13
Kristensen and Sindrup (1978a,b)	22	26	31	79
Hara et al. (1980)	6	4	0	10
Pritchard et al. (1980)	4	1	1	6
Ounsted and Lindsay (1981)	7	0	2	9
Sherwin (1977)	11	3	3	17
Sherwin (1981)	5	2	0	7
Sherwin et al. (1982)	5	2	0	7
Toone et al. (1982a)	4	0	8	12
Parnas et al. (1982)	12	6	7	25
Trimble and Perez (1982)	9	4	4	17
Onuma et al. (1987)	17	5	19	41
Total	146	78	117	341
% of Total	42.8	22.9	34.3	100
% of N	65.2	34.8		

(N) Left + Right (224)

like psychoses with first rank symptoms of Schneider, and seven had a left-sided focus. Perez et al. (1985) used EEG criteria to establish lateralization, and compared the PSE syndrome profiles of patients with left- and right-sided lesions. In their group, eight had consistent left-sided EEG abnormalities, two had bilaterally independent foci, four had right-sided abnormalities, and two had a unilateral focus (one left and one right) in all EEG recordings except their most recent. When the profiles of patients with left-sided abnormalities were compared with those of patients having right-sided abnormalities, two significant differences were noted. The left-sided patients had significantly more nuclear schizophrenia and ideas of reference than right-sided patients (Fig. 9.2).

Sherwin (1977, 1981, 1982) provided evidence from a series of studies carried out in different centres using EEG criteria for the assessment of laterality. In the first report (Sherwin, 1977) of 34 patients with "psychotic-like reactions and aggressivity" 50% had EEGs with localising features, of which 11 were left-sided, 3 were right-sided, and 3 were bilaterally abnormal. In 14 showing temporal horn dilatation, 13 were abnormal on the left side and one was bilaterally abnormal. These findings are in keeping with earlier studies such as that by Larsby and Lindgren (1940), who reported that more than three quarters of "psychiatrically deteriorated" epileptics with ventricular abnormalities revealed left-sided changes.

Seeking better confirmation of laterality, Sherwin (1981, 1982) examined patients who had undergone investigation for temporal lobectomy either at UCLA in California or at INSERM in Paris. From the UCLA group, seven patients were

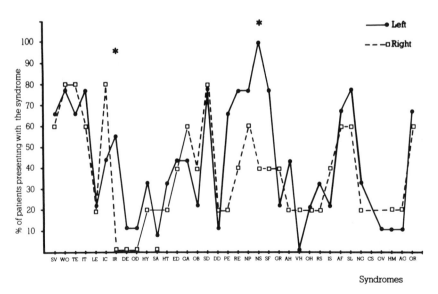

FIG. 9.2. PSE syndrome profiles comparing patients with schizophrenia-like psychoses of epilepsy having a right or left temporal lobe focus. Note the significant association between left temporal lobe epilepsy and nuclei syndrome.

identified as having a paranoid or schizophrenic type psychosis, five of whom had a left temporal lobectomy. In the second sample, seven patients with undifferentiated schizophrenia, paranoid schizophrenia, or hebephrenia were found amongst 80 cases. When the relative frequencies of the left- and right-sided lesions in non-psychotic and psychotic patients were compared, a significant excess of left-sided lesions was found in the psychotic group (five out of seven). In this sample, 46 patients were noted who, for a variety of reasons, did not come to operation. More than half (19 out of 37) of the left-sided nonsurgical cases demonstrated major psychiatric problems, including two cases diagnosed as schizophrenia. In contrast, less than a quarter of the right-sided cases demonstrated such difficulties, and there were no psychotics. Finally, 42 patients were examined who had surgery for other focal epilepsies (frontal, parietal, or occipital lesions) and in these, none had a history of psychosis.

The importance of these surgical studies is that laterality was confirmed by the techniques used for presurgical workup and by improvement in seizures following surgery.

Toone et al. (1982b), in a CT study, noted no laterality findings, although in their psychotic group four schizophrenic patients and one paranoid patient had left-sided abnormalities, and two affective patients had right-sided abnormalities. They further noted that when left-sided and predominantly left-sided abnormalities were compared with right-sided and predominantly right-sided abnormalities, there was an excess of left abnormalities in the psychotic samples (16 vs. 7). For the schizophrenic subgroup the figures were six left and two right. Patients with hallucinations, where a laterality effect was noted, showed a complete absence of right-sided lesions.

The findings with PET and MRI in relation to laterality have been noted above, where hallucinations have been associated with left-sided lesions on MRI (Conlon and Trimble, 1990), and lower left temporal values are noted for metabolic indices in patients with psychosis and temporal lobe epilepsy on PET.

Trimble and colleagues (Perez et al., 1985) extended the argument by noting a more exclusive association between nuclear schizophrenia (confirmed using the PSE) and left hemisphere lesions. Of eleven patients in their series, eight had evidence of left-sided abnormalities, two had a right-sided focus, and one had bilaterally independent foci.

The studies showing laterality in relationship to schizophrenia-like presentations which probably resemble nuclear schizophrenia or in which nuclear schizophrenia has been confirmed using the PSE are shown in Table 9.4. The excess of left-sided lesions is noted, a stronger association than when psychoses generally are examined. This is largely on account of the inclusion in Table 9.3 of patients with affective psychoses which largely, but not exclusively, are noted with right-sided lesions.

The issue of laterality has been examined further by several authors. For Flor-Henry the issue is involvement of the dominant temporal lobe, although Taylor (1975) examines the issue in relationship to sinistrality. Thus, several groups note

TABLE 9.4. *Schizophrenia-like Psychoses of Epilepsy and Laterality of Lesion*

Author	Left	Right	Bilateral	Total
Slater and Beard (1963a,b)	14	10	18	42
Flor-Henry (1969)	9	2	10	21
Taylor (1975)	9	4	0	13
Ounsted and Lindsay (1981)	7	2	0	9
Sherwin (1981)	5	1	0	6
Sherwin et al. (1982)	5	2	0	7
Perez et al. (1985)	8	2	1	11
Total	57	23	29	109
% of Total	52.2	21.1	26.6	100

an excess of sinistrality in relationship to psychosis and temporal lobe epilepsy (Taylor, 1975; Kristensen and Sindrup, 1978a; Toone et al., 1982; Sherwin et al., 1982; Perez and Trimble, 1980b) ranging from 17% to over 70%. Sherwin et al. (1982) specifically examined the relationship to dominance as well as handedness, and noted that it was handedness which was the important issue. Taylor (1975) suggested that sinistrality implied abnormal organisation of cerebral function and did not necessarily specify that there was right hemisphere location for speech in the affected patients. Further, Taylor (1975) and Sherwin et al. (1982) emphasize an interaction between sex, psychosis, and handedness, with an overrepresentation of psychoses in left-handed females.

CONCLUSIONS

The various risk factors associated with the development of the psychoses of epilepsy are shown in Table 9.1, taken from the literature reviewed in this chapter. Certain associations seem relatively clear. For example, the psychoses of epilepsy are overrepresented in patients with epilepsy compared with the general population (see Table 8.4), especially in temporal lobe epilepsy (see Tables 8.5, 8.6). Further, patients with a mediobasal-limbic focus would seem more susceptible (see Table 8.2). When the psychoses are broken down with regard to clinical type, the association between temporal lobe epilepsy and a schizophrenia- or paranoid-like psychosis becomes stronger (see Table 8.11), especially when the left temporal lobe is predominantly affected by the focus (see Table 9.3). In the majority of patients reported in the literature the psychosis follows the epilepsy, the latter beginning in early adolescence (see Table 9.2) with an interval of approximately 11 to 15 years intervening before the onset of the psychosis. Certain subgroups, for example, nuclear schizophrenia as defined by Schneiderian criteria, may be more selective with regard to this variable and to the laterality effect (see Table 9.4).

There are clear associations between a diminished seizure frequency in some patients and the onset of an acute psychosis (as seen in forced normalization) or, more insidiously, with a psychosis emerging as the frequency of seizures diminishes. Psychotic patients are more likely to be left-handed, usually present with complex partial seizures and automatisms and often, but not always, will show evidence of structural pathology, some authors suggesting specific associations, for example, for gangliogliomas (Bruton, 1988).

10

Treatment of Epileptic Psychoses

There are no studies of the treatment of the psychoses of epilepsy, but guidelines have emerged from clinical practice and from animal and human investigations into the effects of psychotropic drugs on the seizure threshold and the EEG. In this chapter, the pharmacology of antipsychotic drugs and lithium will briefly be reviewed prior to a discussion of the relationship between anticonvulsant drugs and psychosis and the role of the latter in treatment. This will be followed by some clinical guidelines for treatment of the epileptic psychoses.

PHARMACOLOGY OF PSYCHOTROPIC AGENTS

Neuroleptic Drugs

Patients who are psychotic require treatments with psychotropic agents that are antipsychotic, and these typically are referred to as major tranquilizers. They naturally fall into four groups: phenothiazines, butyrophenones, thioxanthines and others. The phenothiazines have a tricyclic nucleus, in which different configurations of the side chain lead to alteration of their properties. They include chlorpromazine, thioridazine, and trifluoperazine. Thioxanthines have a similar structure and include clopenthixol, flupenthixol, thiothixene, and related drugs. The butyrophenones, such as haloperidol; and the related diphenylbutylpiperidines, such as pimozide, fluspirilene, and penfluridol have a different chemical structure. Some of this group, for example, penfluridol, are long-acting oral preparations. Finally, the other tranquilizers include reserpine, tetrabenazine, oxypertine, loxapine, clozapine, and the substituted benzamides such as sulpiride.

The distinguishing property of all these drugs is their ability to block dopamine receptors, and clinically they are antipsychotic. In addition they may evoke extrapyramidal symptoms of various types. They all inhibit apomorphine-induced stereotypy and agitation; provoke an acute increase in dopamine turnover with raised

HVA levels in areas of the ventral and dorsal striatum; block the stimulation of dopamine-sensitive adenylate cyclase; and displace receptor binding with H3 dopamine or H3 spiroperidol at postsynaptic dopamine receptor sites (Trimble, 1988). With few exceptions, the ability of these drugs to block the dopamine receptor correlates with their clinical antipsychotic action, particularly blockade of the D-2 receptor. Since the majority readily provoke extrapyramidal effects, it has been suggested that their antipsychotic potential is due to antagonism of dopamine receptors in the mesolimbic or mesocortical areas of the brain, while their motor effects relate to action on the nigrostriatal system.

There are a few drugs that possess minimal potential to evoke extrapyramidal effects, namely, sulpiride, clozapine, and thioridazine. One explanation for this is the anticholinergic potential of some of these drugs which may counteract the tendency to provoke motor disorder. Alternatively, it has been suggested that they preferentially act on dopamine receptors in mesolimbic or mesocortical areas rather than in the striatum. There is limited evidence for a preferential action in mesolimbic areas for these compounds (Leysen and Niemegeers, 1985), and the fact that sulpiride does not possess anticholinergic properties would support the view that the differing clinical effects of these neuroleptics relate to the differential blockade of dopamine receptors. Sulpiride is thought to be a selective D-2 antagonist with a powerful effect on prolactin release which is limited in its ability to provoke motor syndromes in animal models and patients.

Following oral administration, chlorpromazine is well absorbed and metabolised by the liver with peak plasma concentrations occurring in 1 to 3 hours. It has a half-life of 17 hours. Some metabolites such as the sulfoxide, have little pharmacological activity while others, for example, the hydroxyl derivatives, are more potent. It is strongly protein-bound, and preferentially accumulates in the brain with a brain-plasma ratio of about 5:1. After termination of treatment, excretion of the drug or one of its metabolites may continue for several months.

Haloperidol is less rapidly absorbed, maximal concentrations occurring around 5 hours, with a half-life of 13 to 20 hours. It is 90% protein-bound and does not induce its own metabolism. Pimozide has a half-life of over 50 hours, and it is possible to give the drug on less than a once-daily basis. The half-life of sulpiride is 8 hours.

Esterifide drugs, mostly dissolved in oil, are given intramuscularly and released over a varying period of time, up to about 4 weeks. They include the decanoate preparations of haloperidol, fluphenazine, flupenthixol, and clopenthixol. These drugs provoke the same incidence of extrapyramidal problems as do oral preparations, although the onset of these may be more rapid.

In general, the extrapyramidal syndromes form into two groups, the acute and the less acute. In practice, some admixture of symptoms is seen and the division may not be so clear. The acute disorders include dystonias, akathisia, akinesia, and parkinsonism. The chronic ones are mainly tardive dystonia and tardive dyskinesia. The biochemistry of these disorders is still unclear, although theories generally relate to alteration of dopamine activity within basal ganglia structures. In treatment, particular attention should be paid to akathisia, which affects up to 50% of patients on these prescriptions. It is characterised by a subjective sense of restlessness and presents as motor hyperactivity with shifting posture and inability to sit or stay still for more than a few moments. It thus resembles agitation, and may be mistaken for the agitation of an affective disorder or psychosis. It may be associated with orofacial dyskinesia. It usually responds to a reduction of dose or to the administration of anticholinergic or benzodiazepine drugs.

Lithium

The other major psychotropic drug used in the management of psychoses is lithium carbonate, which was introduced for the treatment of manic-depressive illness in 1949. Following ingestion it is rapidly absorbed, peak concentrations occurring in 1 to 2 hours, with a half-life of approximately 24 hours. It is mainly excreted in the urine, thus patients with renal disease readily become intoxicated. Since it is reabsorbed with sodium into the proximal renal tubules, any drug that leads to a negative sodium balance such as a diuretic, will lead to increased retention of lithium. This also occurs with alteration of diet, heavy sweating, and diseases that reduce sodium intake.

Its mode of action is unknown in spite of its widespread use, but it does reduce the sodium content of the brain, increase central 5-HT [5-hydroxytryptamine (serotonin)] synthesis and noradrenaline turnover, and increase platelet 5-HT uptake (Coppen et al., 1980).

Its main indication is in the management of bipolar disorders, although it is now known to be useful in the management of recurrent unipolar affective disorder. It is also used in the acute treatment of affective disorder, especially mania, when it is often started in combination with a major tranquilizer or carbamazepine. Its toxic effects are shown in Table 10.1.

The incidence of side effects is minimised by regular serum level monitoring, and it has been suggested that levels below 1.5 μ/mol per litre are relatively safe. However, severe toxicity has been described at lower levels, and coexisting medication such as phenytoin, carbamazepine, or haloperidol may be related to this. Ibuprofen, indomethacin, mefenamic acid, diclofenac, and piroxicam inhibit lithium excretion and diuretics cause lithium retention, increasing serum levels. Patients with cardiac or renal disease or those in situations that lead to interference with the clearance of lithium need regular monitoring.

Prior to starting therapy it is customary to assess renal, hepatic, and thyroid function, the latter since lithium has been associated with goitre or even advanced myxoedema in chronic therapy. However, lithium decreases thyroxine and T3 levels and increases thyroid stimulating hormone (TSH) which leads to abnormalities of thyroid function tests in the absence of clinical hypothyroidism. If lithium maintenance becomes essential in the presence of hypothyroidism, then supplementary thyroxine treatment can be given.

One of the most common side effects relates to alteration of renal function with

TABLE 10.1. *Toxic Effects of Lithium*

Neuropsychiatric	Drowsiness
	Confusion
	Psychomotor retardation
	Restlessness
	Stupor
	Headache
	Weakness
	Tremor
	Ataxia
	Myasthenia gravis syndrome
	Peripheral neuropathy
	Choreoathetoid movements
	Dysarthria
	Dysgeusia
	Blurred vision
	Seizures
	Dizziness, vertigo
	Impaired short-term memory and concentration
Gastrointestinal	Anorexia, nausea, vomiting
	Diarrhoea
	Dry mouth, metallic taste
	Weight gain
Renal	Microtubular lesions
	Impairment of renal concentrating capacity
Cardiovascular	Low blood pressure
	ECG changes
Endocrine	Myxoedema
	Hyperthyroidism
	Hyperparathyroidism
Other	Polyuria and polydipsia
	Glycosuria
	Hypercalciuria
	Rashes

polyuria and polydipsia. Urinary concentrating ability is impaired, which may be exacerbated by combination of lithium with neuroleptics. The polyuria may result in compensatory increases in antidiuretic hormone secretion, although occasionally a picture of nephrogenic diabetes insipidus is seen. This is in contrast to the effects of carbamazepine, which has been used to treat diabetes insipidus. However, when used in combination, carbamazepine will not override the lithium-induced diabetes insipidus.

Severe lithium intoxication may lead to an organic brain syndrome with hyperactive reflexes, seizures, and tremor, and on occasions unilateral neurological abnormalities have been reported which may be interpreted as an alternative neurological diagnosis.

ANTICONVULSANT DRUGS

Obviously, most patients with epileptic psychosis will be receiving one or more anticonvulsant drugs. The pharmacology and mode of action of the more widely used compounds are briefly discussed. A table of the anticonvulsant drugs currently in use is shown in Table 10.2.

In general, the older barbiturate-related compounds and phenytoin are gradually being replaced by newer drugs, especially carbamazepine and sodium valproate. Phenytoin is highly plasma-bound and cleared by hepatic metabolism. Varying serum levels may be noted amongst different patients on the same dose, and small increments in prescription can lead to rapidly escalating serum levels on account of its zero-order pharmacokinetics. In spite of its long use, its mechanism of action is unknown, although it does alter transport mechanisms regulating sodium and calcium flux across neuronal membranes, leading to a decrease in intracellular sodium and calcium concentrations. This leads to a blockade of neurotransmitter release, limiting the potential for high-frequency neuronal discharges. It is a membrane

TABLE 10.2. *Some Anticonvulsant Drugs in Current Use*

Drug name (Trade name)	Indications
Carbamazepine (Tegretol)	Seizures: generalised simple partial complex partial secondary generalised
Clobazam (Frisium)	Seizures: generalised simple partial complex partial secondary generalised
Clonazepam (Klonopin, Rivotril)	Myoclonic epilepsy
Ethosuximide (Zarontin)	Seizures: generalised absence
Phenobarbitone	Seizures: generalised simple partial
Phenytoin (Dilantin, Epanutin)	Seizures: generalised simple partial complex partial
Primidone (Mysoline)	Seizures: generalised simple partial complex partial
Valproic acid (Depakene, Epilim)	Myoclonic epilepsy Seizures: generalised absence simple partial complex partial
Vigabatrin (Sabril)	Seizures: generalised partial secondary generalised

stabilizer and also possesses some benzodiazepine binding properties and thus has some influence on the GABA receptor, particularly at higher concentrations.

Primidone is partially converted to phenobarbitone, although the primidone component itself probably exerts independent anticonvulsant activity. The mechanism of action of phenobarbitone remains unclear but it, too, interacts with the GABA receptor enhancing GABAergic inhibition. It also influences the transcellular transport of sodium, calcium, and potassium ions, influencing the neurotransmitter release of GABA and excitatory amino acids such as glutamate and aspartate.

Carbamazepine is structurally related to the tricyclic antidepressants and has a mode of action different from phenytoin and phenobarbitone. Its biochemical actions include partial agonism of adenosine receptors; increased firing of the locus ceruleus; and decreases in CSF somatostatin and HVA accumulation after probenecid (Post and Uhde, 1986; Post et al., 1986). Further, in animal models, carbamazepine has been shown to be more effective than other anticonvulsants in inhibiting seizures developed from amygdala kindling, suggesting some limbic system selectivity for the drug (Albright and Burnham, 1980). It inhibits sodium channel influx and interacts with peripheral benzodiazepine receptors and the GABA-B receptor (Pippenger, 1989).

Ever since its introduction for the management of epilepsy, carbamazepine has been reported to have some psychotropic properties, and recently its use as a mood stabilizer in manic-depressive illness has been widely investigated and reviewed (Post et al., 1989). Carbamazepine appears to be as effective as conventional neuroleptics in the management of acute mania, especially in patients who are severely ill, show intense dysphoria, rapid cycling, and have a negative family history for affective disorder. It is used in the prophylaxis of bipolar affective disorder, either alone or in combination with lithium. Further, in uncontrolled studies, moderate or marked clinical improvements have been reported with carbamazepine as adjunctive therapy in schizophrenia. The precise symptoms which respond remain unclear, various authors reporting significant improvements in different aspects of the syndrome (Post and Uhde, 1986).

In the management of epilepsy, carbamazepine has become the drug of choice for the management of complex partial seizures, but is also used in the control of aggression and episodic dyscontrol.

Sodium valproate (valproic acid) is thought to be a GABA agonist. It also reduces sodium and potassium conductance reducing the excitability of nerve membranes. However, its mode of action is unknown at the present time. As with carbamazepine, there is recent evidence suggesting it may have mood-stabilising properties (Post et al., 1989) which, however, is less secure.

The role of benzodiazepines in the management of epilepsy has been largely restricted to acute use in status epilepticus, but a number, including clonazepam and clobazam, have found value as oral therapy. The latter is a nonsedative 1,5-benzodiazepine which has recently become accepted as adjunctive therapy in difficult-to-treat children and adult patients.

Vigabatrin has just been introduced for clinical practice. It is an irreversible inhibitor of GABA-transaminase, and increases brain GABA as a consequence. It has been used in patients with difficult-to-control seizures of a variety of types.

The chronic side effects of anticonvulsants are legion, and are outlined in Table 10.3.

Neuropsychiatric effects, in particular of phenytoin, include an encephalopathy and deterioration of intellectual function while apathy, depression, dysphoria, irritability, and occasionally hyperactivity are associated with barbiturates. Chronic dyskinesias are occasionally seen, and an acute dystonic reaction has been noted with carbamazepine. Sodium valproate has been associated with liver failure in a small number of young patients, and produces a reversible alopecia and weight gain.

Psychoses have been reported in association with most anticonvulsants, largely as anecdotal reports. Included are phenytoin, primidone, carbamazepine, vigabatrin, and sodium valproate, the latter provoking in some patients an encephalopathy leading to profound stupor. The psychoses associated with ethosuximide and vigabatrin are often seizure-related, occurring as a consequence of forced normalisation or as postictal psychoses associated with clustering (Sander et al., 1991).

TABLE 10.3. *Chronic Toxic Effects of Some Anticonvulsant Drugs*

Site	Effects
Nervous system	Cerebellar atrophy
	Peripheral neuropathy
	Encephalopathy
	Other mental symptoms
Haemopoietic system	Folic acid deficiency
	Neonatal coagulation defects
Skeletal system	Metabolic bone disease
	Vitamin D deficiency
Connective tissue	Gum hypertrophy
	Facial skin changes
	Wound healing impairment
	Dupuytren's contracture
Skin	Hirsutism, alopecia
	Pigmentation
	Acne
Liver	Enzyme induction
Endocrine system	Pituitary-adrenal dysfunction
	Thyroid-parathyroid change
	Hyperglycaemia (diabetogenic)
Metabolic disorders	Vitamin B_6 deficiency
	Heavy metal disorders
Immune system	Lymphotoxicity
	Lymphadenopathy
	Systemic lupus erythematosus
	Antinuclear antibodies
	Immunoglobulin changes
	Immunosuppression

Recently the dangers of unwanted polytherapy in epilepsy have been emphasised, and it is generally accepted that newly diagnosed patients should be treated with monotherapy. It has been shown that upward of 80% of new patients, with appropriate serum level monitoring and adequate serum levels, will be satisfactorily controlled. It is not clear that the addition of a second drug will lead to the better management of seizures in those who continue to have attacks, with certain exceptions. Patients often improve, both from the point of view of their psychological function and also their seizure frequency, when unbridled polytherapy is rationalised to monotherapy (Thompson and Trimble, 1982).

PHARMACOKINETIC INTERACTIONS

Patients with epileptic psychoses are likely to be treated with either a major tranquilizer or lithium, and the interactions between these drugs and anticonvulsants are outlined in Tables 10.4 and 10.5.

It can be seen that the number of interactions which have been investigated is limited. In general, there are anecdotal reports that phenothiazines can precipitate phenytoin intoxication, and there is evidence that chlorpromazine and thioridazine increase serum phenytoin levels, probably by inhibiting its metabolism (Perucca et al., 1985). In practice, however, many patients tolerate the combination of a phenothiazine with an anticonvulsant without any obvious change in phenytoin or phenobarbitone levels (Linnoila et al., 1980). In view of the possibilities of idiosyncratic reactions, it is probably wise to monitor serum anticonvulsant levels following the initiation of these drugs, especially if a deterioration of behaviour occurs.

The enzyme-inducing activity of the majority of anticonvulsants stimulates the metabolism of neuroleptics, leading to reduced levels (Curry et al., 1970). Since sodium valproate does not appear to induce hepatic enzymes, interference with serum levels is likely to be less with this anticonvulsant. Phenobarbitone is reported to increase the urinary excretion of chlorpromazine (Forrest et al., 1970) and carbamazepine decreases haloperidol levels by up to 60% (Jann et al., 1985). Data with lithium are scarce, but the addition of phenytoin has been reported to provoke lithium toxicity (MacCallum, 1980).

TABLE 10.4. *Some Interactions Between Anticonvulsants*

Anticonvulsant	Effect on phenytoin levels
Sulthiame	↑
Diazepam, clonazepam	↓
Carbamazepine[a]	↓
Phenobarbitone	↓
Valproate[b]	↑ (free levels)

[a]Carbamazepine reduces the serum concentration of phenytoin and vice versa.

[b]Sodium valproate displaces phenytoin from its protein binding sites, increasing the unbound fraction of phenytoin.

TABLE 10.5. *Some Interactions Between Anticonvulsants and Other Drugs*

Drugs whose effects are reduced with anticonvulsants	Drugs which may induce anticonvulsant toxicity
Warfarin and coumarin anticonvulsants	Isoniazid
Cortisol, dexamethasone and prednisolone	Dicoumarol
Contraceptive pill	Disulfiram
Vitamin D	Chloramphenicol
Phenylbutazone	Imipramine
Antidepressants	Chlorpromazine
Chlorpromazine	Chlorpheniramine
Haloperidol	Erythromycin
Digoxin	Methylphenidate
Diazepam	Lithium

PSYCHOTROPIC DRUGS AND SEIZURE THRESHOLD

Animal Studies

It is well known that many psychotropic drugs lower the seizure threshold and can provoke convulsions (Trimble, 1978). In laboratory studies some comparative data are available. Thus, Meldrum et al. (1975) compared the effect of haloperidol and pimozide on the epileptic threshold of the photosensitive baboon, Papio papio. Both drugs led to an increase in spike-wave and slow-wave activity, although less enhancement of the myoclonic epileptic responses was seen following pimozide. Oliver et al. (1982) used spike activity in perfused guinea pig hippocampal slices to assess the seizure potential of several neuroleptic drugs. In this model, pimozide showed few changes, the maximum increase in neuronal excitability being shown by haloperidol, thioridazine, and chlorpromazine. Combinations of chlorpromazine and haloperidol were particularly effective at increasing seizure activity.

Lithium appeared to have only minimal proconvulsant activity using models of kindled seizures (Clifford et al., 1985).

Human Studies

The effects of chlorpromazine on the EEG are similar to those of tricyclic antidepressants, and it was used as an EEG-activating agent in doses between 25 mg and 100 mg intravenously (Kiloh et al., 1961). Chlorpromazine and related phenothiazines provoke increased slow-wave activity with synchronization of the EEG. Even small IV doses provoke a marked increase of paroxysmal dysrhythmic activity, sharp waves, and focal spike waves when given to epileptic patients, especially those with 3 cps spike-wave activity on the EEG (Itil, 1970). Similar findings have been noted for related compounds such as promazine and thioridazine, although the latter induces less synchronization, and appears less provocative than chlorpromazine. Significant activation was not described following perphenazine, or following long-acting fluphenazine (Itil, 1970). The thioxanthines appear similar to phenothiazines, and haloperidol activates epileptic potentials in a similar manner.

NEUROLEPTIC DRUGS AND SEIZURES: CLINICAL STUDIES

The facility of neuroleptic drugs to provoke epileptic seizures in patients with or without epilepsy is well known (Logothetis, 1967). The evidence for this is largely from anecdotal studies, although examination of EEG patterns reflects this potential. Thus, in the normal human EEG, a tendency to synchronization with increased slower frequencies and an increase in amplitude, often more prominent in temporal areas, occurs following chlorpromazine. Preexisting EEG abnormalities of a diffuse or focal nature are accentuated (Jorgensen and Wulff, 1958).

Epileptic seizures have been observed in patients receiving oral phenothiazines, in patients with preexisting paroxysmal epileptiform EEG patterns, and there are several reports of patients in whom phenothiazines have precipitated seizures with no prior history of convulsions (Logothetis, 1967). In one review of the literature, Logothetis (1967) noted that the percentage of nonepileptic subjects having convulsions varied, on low to moderate amounts of chlorpromazine (up to 1 g per day), from 0.3% to 5% (mean 2.1%). With larger doses, figures of up to 50% had been noted. Seizures tended to occur with larger amounts of phenothiazines, either shortly after the initiation of the drug or following a sudden increase in dosage. There was evidence that organic brain dysfunction was associated with a higher frequency of seizures, and in this series chlorpromazine was the drug most implicated, although it was the drug most commonly prescribed. Other reviewers, however, also suggest chlorpromazine to be the most epileptogenic (Remick and Fine, 1979; Mendez et al., 1986).

There are clinical reports of seizures occurring with the majority of phenothiazines, although thioridazine, which has strong anticholinergic properties, has been recommended for the management of behaviour disorders in epileptic patients (Kamm and Mandel, 1967). Fluphenazine (particularly given intramuscularly as the decanoate preparation) and butyrophenones are generally considered to be safer.

The major tranquilizer, itself, is only one variable which relates to precipitation of seizures, other factors having been investigated by Toone and Fenton (1977). Information from case histories of 41 patients who experienced seizures thought to be related to psychotropic drug use was compared with a control group. The seizure patients were more commonly first-born children and had a history of postnatal brain damage. During the first week preceding the seizure there had been a marked increase in drug prescription. These data identify preexisting organic damage and initiation of drug or dose change as important factors. Other studies have noted a family history of epilepsy in nonepileptic patients prone to convulsions (Betts et al., 1968).

Lithium, which in animal models has a proconvulsant effect (Clifford et al., 1985), is also associated with seizures, sometimes within the therapeutic range (Demers et al., 1970).

A summary of the experimental and clinical data would therefore suggest that there is a spectrum of convulsant potential of the neuroleptic drugs, with the phenothiazines (especially chlorpromazine) being maximally convulsant. Drugs of the butyrophenone group are less likely to provoke seizures. Experimental data would suggest that pimozide has the least convulsant potential, although reliable comparative clinical data are not available.

TREATMENT OF THE ICTAL AND INTERICTAL PSYCHOSES

Ictal Psychoses

The management of the ictal and interictal psychoses are different. Ictal psychoses, directly related to the acute electrical disturbances of the seizure, clearly require better control of seizures for prevention of further episodes. In particular, prevention of seizure clusters seem important in a subgroup of patients in whom these precede an acute psychotic episode. One cause for such clusters is noncompliance, and occasionally patients with an evolving psychosis stop their drugs under the influence of delusions of instruction from some third party, such as a deity.

Several studies show a high incidence of noncompliance in patients with epilepsy. For example, Gibberd et al. (1970) quoted a figure of 42% failing to take treatment as prescribed, some studies (Kutt et al., 1966) showing even higher rates. The reasons for noncompliance are multiple. Peterson et al. (1982), in a study of 101 teenage and adult patients, noted only 50% to be compliant in taking their anticonvulsant medication correctly. The epileptic variables that related to compliance included more frequent generalised tonic-clonic seizures, patients more worried about health, perceiving no barriers to obtaining regular care and medication, and noticing the effects of missing medication. While the first two of these seem predictable, the third is worthy of much consideration in terms of improved doctor-patient relationships and the facility with which patients with epilepsy can get access to people who know about their disorder, its complications and management.

Peterson et al. also noted that important determinants of noncompliance were inconvenience of taking medications and forgetfulness. It is still a fact that many patients receive polypharmacy when, as noted, seizure control may be just as good using monotherapy. Since compliance is adversely affected by polytherapy, attempts to get such patients with seizure clusters on a well-rationalised monotherapy regime can be worthwhile. Paying attention to timing of dose is also important, and there are few anticonvulsants that need to be given three to four times a day. To ask schoolchildren and adolescents to take a dose of medicine at lunchtime, or officeworkers to take one at teatime is often incompatible, not only with their need to appear "normal," but also with any memory impairments they may be suffering from, either as a consequence of the seizure disorder or their medications. Twice-daily regimes are best prescribed in the morning and at night, and once-daily regimes, if compatible with the control of seizures, on a nighttime basis.

Patients who have ictally related psychoses and complex partial seizures are most appropriately treated by carbamazepine monotherapy. Patients with generalised absence seizure status require sodium valproate or ethosuximide, and patients with mixed types of seizures may be prescribed more than one drug on a rational basis dependent upon seizure classification.

The question of surgery for patients with psychoses is discussed in Chapter 7 where it was noted that, in the majority of centres, psychotic patients tend to be excluded from this treatment. However, if the psychosis is seen to be driven by seizures which are clearly from one or another temporal lobe, and if surgery is an option for the seizures, then this must be given careful consideration. Thus, discrete episodes of peri-ictal psychosis should not be seen as a contraindication to surgical intervention, but postoperatively there may be a risk for the development of a postoperative psychosis. Psychiatric follow-up will be required.

Sometimes during the psychotic episode, antipsychotic medications are required. Haloperidol or pimozide are preferable. They may need to be given intravenously or intramuscularly, especially if the patient is noncompliant, although oral administration is better. Doses of 0.5 to 10 mg of haloperidol (2 to 40 mg of pimozide) may be required at regular intervals initially, although when any acute disturbance of behaviour is controlled, the doses needed will be less. It is important that patients with only ictally related psychoses are not kept on these medications chronically, and when the psychosis has resolved they should be slowly withdrawn.

Interictal Psychoses

In contrast, the interictal psychoses should be managed very much as psychiatric disorders in the absence of epilepsy. Manic-depressive psychosis is treated with lithium, although the antimanic properties of carbamazepine suggest that it would be logical to treat patients with bipolar disorders and epilepsy on carbamazepine monotherapy if possible. Individual episodes of mania may require a major tranquilizer such as a phenothiazine or butyrophenone, while the depressive phases will require antidepressant therapy or ECT.

Choice of antidepressant is difficult since the majority of non-MAOI (monoamine oxidase inhibitor) antidepressants lower the seizure threshold and may provoke seizures clinically (Trimble, 1978). Drugs particularly implicated include maprotiline, mianserin hydrochloride, amitriptyline hydrochloride, and imipramine hydrochloride, some of the widely used antidepressants. Even the newer selective 5-HT uptake inhibitors are not free from the potential to provoke seizures. One group has reported that doxepin leads to improved seizure frequency in depressed epileptic patients (Ojemann et al., 1983).

Whichever antidepressant is chosen, it should be noted that pharmacokinetic interactions are of importance. Patients receiving anticonvulsant drugs tend to have lower antidepressant levels than those not on such drugs, although idiosyncratic anticonvulsant toxicity has been reported for several antidepressants of the tricyclic and nontricyclic varieties (Perucca et al., 1985). Deterioration of behaviour following prescription of such psychotropics, therefore, requires immediate attention to the alteration of the behaviour state and measurements of serum levels of the anticonvulsant drugs to assess if toxicity may have occurred. The fact that serum antidepressant levels may be low means that higher oral doses than usual will need to be given before a clinical response may occur. This will increase the chances of provoking a seizure.

Whichever antidepressant is used, in patients with epilepsy the depressive episodes associated with bipolar disorder and acute unipolar depressive psychosis may be short lived. It is sometimes more judicious to withhold antidepressant treatment and avoid the risk of increasing seizure frequency and causing unwarranted pharmacokinetic interactions. In general, rationalising polytherapy, particularly attempting carbamazepine monotherapy, is shown to have an antidepressant effect in epileptic patients with depressive symptoms (Thompson and Trimble, 1982).

Electroconvulsive therapy is not contraindicated in patients with epilepsy, and should always be used when suicide is a real danger or in cases of severe paranoid agitation, particularly if the patient's seizure frequency appears to have declined prior to the onset of the depressive or psychotic episode. The most appropriate method for administering ECT is with unilateral placement of electrodes to the nondominant hemisphere, and a course of 8 to 12 treatments, given twice a week, will usually resolve the clinical problem. Care should be taken that the patient does not switch into mania, in which case antimanic therapy would be required.

Paranoid and schizophrenia-like states also need to be evaluated in terms of their onset in relationship to seizure frequency. Thus, as noted, several authors have hinted that psychosis can occur when seizure frequency is declining, another manifestation of the antagonism of von Meduna and Landolt (see Chapter 5). In these patients, or in those who stop having seizures completely in association with the onset of the psychosis, a neuroleptic medication which increases the seizure threshold may be the most logical prescription. Thus, chlorpromazine would be a clinical choice. Depending on the severity of the presentation, the doses prescribed will be equivalent to that of psychiatric conditions in the absence of epilepsy, ranging from 100 to 1000 mg per day. Where a clear biological link appears to exist between the suppression of seizures and the development of the psychosis, ECT should be considered necessary if the patient is extremely agitated, very paranoid, or is suicidal. In patients in whom seizure frequency has diminished when they are psychotic, particularly if the psychosis is chronic, careful consideration should be given to the possibility of reducing anticonvulsant therapy even to the extent of permitting seizures to occur if this is beneficial.

Where patients with epilepsy have no alteration of seizure frequency, or where psychosis occurs in a setting of increased seizure frequency, a neuroleptic drug less likely to precipitate seizures is probably more appropriate. Here butyrophenones would be the drugs of choice, either haloperidol or pimozide, in gradually increasing doses. Sulpiride would appear to be a reasonable alternative. The animal data would suggest that combinations of chlorpromazine and haloperidol are best avoided. For longer term management, intramuscular preparations such as flupenthixol decanoate can be useful, being given once a month or once every 3 weeks, often in the absence of additional oral neuroleptic therapy.

As in all psychiatric problems, psychopharmacological management alone is not sufficient. Although the role of psychotherapy in the management of psychotic conditions has not proven of any substantial value, it is important to acknowledge that epileptic patients with psychosis bear the burden of epilepsy in addition to their psychosis. Patients with intermittent psychotic states are often perplexed and embarrassed by what has happened to them while psychotic, and fear further continuing bouts. Patients with continuous psychosis required the skills of paramedical intervention, and the full resources of community care may need to be brought to them in order to help them rehabilitate and to assist their families in coping with their difficulties. In many patients with chronic psychoses of epilepsy the preservation of affect and lack of personality disintegration over years sustain them well in their communities, and enable many such patients to live within their families or to be married. Bringing such support to them is of importance in maintaining their lives in the community and preventing their recurrent admission to hospital. Further, in a good family environment with adequate medical facilities and follow-up care, patient compliance will tend to be good; deterioration of an otherwise delicate situation, induced by poor compliance and leading to more seizures and exacerbations of psychopathology, with loss of control by the family and the physician, may hopefully be avoided.

11

ECT, Seizures, Epilepsy, and Psychosis

CONVULSIVE THERAPY

As noted in Chapter 1 and explored further in Chapter 5, there is a long history to the antithetical relationship between psychosis and seizures. Although convulsive therapy was initially carried out using camphor for the treatment of schizophrenia, electrical means of inducing a seizure are now routinely used. The clinical use of ECT has been established for many years, but recently several double-blind controlled trials of its efficacy have been carried out (see for review Crow and Johnstone, 1986), the majority in affective disorder. Nonetheless, trials against simulated ECT have also reported benefits in schizophrenia (Taylor and Fleminger, 1980).

A consistent predictor of response in studies of affective disorder has been the presence of delusions. There are eight studies that address this issue (Janicak et al., 1989). For example, the prospective study of Crow and colleagues (Crow and Johnstone, 1986) examined real versus simulated ECT in 70 patients with major depression. After 4 weeks of treatment, 10 psychotically depressed patients had a 78% change of score compared with 68% in those without psychosis. One of the conclusions of the investigators was "the most salient predictor of response to real ECT is probably the presence of delusions." Janicak et al., (1989) compared the effect of ECT in 13 psychotic to 20 nonpsychotic patients and noted a greater reduction in depressive rating scales in psychotic depressives after an average of 9.2 treatments.

There is then evidence that the seizure of ECT not only resolves affective disorder, but is particularly helpful in the presence of psychosis. The question arises as to the mechanism of action of ECT that may be related to these effects. Unfortunately, the mechanism of action of ECT is not known. It seems clear that changes in brain function evolve over time, reflected in the usual practice of administering therapy two or three times a week. The antidepressant effect is directly related to the seizure activity (Ottosson, 1960), cumulative seizure duration being an important variable.

Maletzky (1978) estimated that if the total seizure time was less than 201 seconds, no response was noted, while most patients responded after 1,000 seconds.

A number of biochemical and electrophysiological changes following electroconvulsive shock (ECS) in animal models have been shown. There is down regulation of beta adrenergic receptor sites (Bergstrom and Kellar, 1979) consistent with most other antidepressant treatments, and changes appear to parallel the clinical effects observed in patients over time. ECS also enhances the synaptic availability of catecholamines, increasing the activity of tyrosine hydrolase, the rate-limiting enzyme for catecholamine biosynthesis (Musacchio et al., 1969) and reducing the uptake of noradrenaline into synaptic preparations (Hendley and Welch, 1975). ECS enhances behavioural responses to 5-HT, probably due to an increase in the number of $5\text{-}HT_2$ receptors (Vetulani et al., 1981).

Other effects that may have relevance include enhanced dopamine-related behaviours with repeated ECS, enhanced GABA activity, and also effects on opiate responses. Thus, ECS enhances behavioural and neuroendocrine responses to dopamine agonists (Grahame-Smith et al., 1978) and increases the number of frontocortical GABA-B receptors (Lloyd et al., 1985b). Chronic ECS enhances opioid receptor binding (Belenky et al., 1984).

It is difficult to see how these biochemical effects interlink with the antipsychotic action of ECT, although some of these actions have been replicated in human studies. For example, a course of ECT is followed by an increased growth hormone response to apomorphine, consistent with increasing dopamine agonism (Costain et al., 1982). ECT seems to have a consistent effect in Parkinson's disease (for review see Faber and Trimble, 1991), and changes in serum prolactin occur after both epileptic seizures and those induced by convulsive therapy (Trimble, 1978), with a tendency towards diminished prolactin release with successive treatments. One group has shown that CSF 5-HIAA and HVA increase significantly following a course of ECT, suggesting increased turnover of both serotonin and dopamine (Rudorfer et al., 1988).

It is unclear how increasing the turnover of such monoamines could lead to an antipsychotic effect as the bulk of evidence suggests that increasing dopaminergic activity leads to an increase in the chances of developing psychosis, and most effective antipsychotics reduce dopamine function.

An interesting feature of ECS and ECT is that they are anticonvulsant in action. Thus, single and multiple ECS in animal models lead to anticonvulsant effects against amygdala kindled seizures (Post et al., 1986a). CSF collected from animals with such elevated thresholds, when transferred to the ventricular space of untreated animals, confers on the untreated animals an elevated threshold (Long and Tortella, 1984). There is also evidence from human studies that ECT increases the seizure threshold (Sackeim et al., 1987).

These data are interesting in the light of the growing knowledge that some anticonvulsants possess antipsychotic and, in particular, antimanic properties (see Chapter 10).

There is speculation that the behavioural effect of seizures may be related to opioid effects (Nakajima et al., 1989). Thus, some opioid peptides have anticonvulsant action, and peptides are released by a seizure. It is conceivable that some released peptides also influence behaviour, although generally, authors who have written about this are seeking mechanisms for explanation of the improved affective state of patients undergoing ECT rather than seeking links between seizures and psychosis. Indeed, biochemical evidence to date does not reveal the underlying mechanism of the antipsychotic effect of seizures and does not shed light on why patients with seizures should, in certain circumstances, undergo resolution of an epileptic psychosis. The possibility that it is nonspecific should be entertained. Thus, rather as cardiac conversion in atrial fibrillation, the seizure may "reset" a disturbed neurochemical/neurophysiological environment—similar to Hill's theory of homoeostasis (Hill, 1956, see Chapter 5). Nonetheless, the relevance of the ECT effect on psychosis cannnot be underestimated for further exploring links between seizures and psychosis, as is revealed through antagonisms between the symptoms of psychoses and seizures, well-documented over the years.

SCHIZOPHRENIA AND THE TEMPORAL LOBES

One of the persistent themes of this book has been that patients with temporal lobe epilepsy are more likely to develop psychopathology, especially if the abnormal electrical activity derives from medial temporal structures affecting the limbic system. The phenomenology of these psychoses often involves schizophrenia-like or paranoid states, and only specific differences, for example, the relative maintenance of warm affect and lack of motor symptoms, distinguishes schizophrenia from the schizophrenia-like psychoses of epilepsy. An important consequence of this is that the schizophrenia-like psychoses of epilepsy are a biological model for at least some forms of schizophrenia, notably those presenting with similar phenomenology. Included would be patients with positive symptom (Crow's type 1) schizophrenia, and an emphasis in some of the epilepsy studies has been on the presence of first rank symptoms. If the biological model has validity, and if the temporal lobes are involved in the pathogenesis of the schizophrenia-like psychoses of epilepsy, then it is in the temporal lobes in particular that one should seek changes in schizophrenia, in the absence of epilepsy. The evidence that limbic system structures are involved in schizophrenia comes from several areas, but notably from neuropathological studies, neurophysiological investigations, and radiological data. This literature is now reviewed.

NEUROPATHOLOGICAL DATA

As already noted, von Meduna was impressed by the apparent opposite pathologies of schizophrenia and epilepsy. In schizophrenia there was loss of neurones and no glial reaction, while in epilepsy there was only slight loss of neurones and more massive glial reactions. However, interesting regional differences have only become apparent with more recent studies.

Limbic system abnormalities in brains from schizophrenics were shown by Nieto and Escobar (1972). They detected gliosis in the periventricular and midbrain areas, including the hypothalamus, thalamus, septal area, and periaqueductal grey area. However, the hippocampus was also affected. Similar data, also using glial stains, were reported by Stevens (1982) on a series of patients hospitalized prior to use of neuroleptic medication. Gliosis was maximal in periventricular, periaqueductal, and basal forebrain regions. Nuclei involved included the thalamus, hypothalamus, septal, bed nucleus of the stria terminalis, substantia innominata, and nucleus accumbens. Changes were also noted in the amygdala. Neurone loss or infarction was seen in the globus pallidus, and several cases showed disruption of fibre bundles traversing the periaqueductal region, such as the fornix and stria terminalis. Stevens interpreted these data as compatible with evidence of third and lateral ventricular enlargement in schizophrenia, the pathology affecting predominantly limbic structures.

Bogerts and colleagues (Bogerts et al., 1985: Falkai et al., 1988), in a series of studies of schizophrenia on brains from the Vogt collection (from patients who never received ECT, insulin, or neuroleptic treatment) reported reduced volume in five areas. The greatest was the parahippocampal gyrus, others being the hippocampus, amygdala, globus pallidus, and periventricular region. The inferior horn of the lateral ventricle also showed enlargement. In a more specific study of the entorhinal region they noted a significant volume reduction in schizophrenics versus controls with a 37% reduction of neurones, although no excess of gliosis was reported. They believed their data suggested a developmental hypoplasia of medial temporal structures in schizophrenia rather than an ongoing pathological process which would have been associated with gliosis. In a comparison of their findings in schizophrenia with those of brains from patients with Huntington's chorea and Parkinson's disease, it was the hippocampal changes that were the most striking (Bogerts et al., 1983).

Stevens (1986) reported on a clinicopathological correlation of Bogerts' data and noted that pallidum changes were more often associated with negativism and catalepsy, while thought disorder was associated with pathology in the parahippocampal gyrus and enlargement of the inferior horn of the lateral ventricles. Hallucinations and paranoia were seen with amygdala and hippocampal pathology.

Further data in relation to hippocampal pathology in schizophrenia has been reported by Kovelman and Scheibel (1984). They reported pyramidal cell disorganization in two separate groups of brains from schizophrenic patients, again suggestive of disruption at an early stage of CNS development. The pathology occurred throughout the Ammon's horn but mainly involved interface zones; between prosubiculum and CA1, between CA1 and CA2, and between CA2 and CA3.

Hippocampal pathology in schizophrenia has more recently been studied by Jeste and Lohr (1989); most patients had never received neuroleptics, the brains being taken from the Yakovlev collection. Using semiautomated image analysis, they computed volume and pyramidal cell density in the hippocampus. They reported that sections from schizophrenic patients consistently had the lowest volume and pyramidal cell density in comparison to nonschizophrenic patients and normal controls. In their study, differences were greatest in the left CA3 and CA4 regions. They attributed this to possible abnormal prenatal migration of neuroblasts into the hippocampal primordium. The relevance of CA4 abnormalities to the development of psychosis will be discussed later, but it is of note that some of the negative pathological studies have not studied this region; for example, Christison et al. (1989), who were unable to find abnormal array patterns in CA1 regions from the midhippocampus of schizophrenic patients.

The question of the association of developmental abnormalities with these pathological changes has been followed further by Jakob and Beckmann (1989) and Crow and colleagues (Brown et al., 1986; Crow et al., 1989). Jakob and Beckmann examined the brains of 76 chronic schizophrenic patients matched with controls. Twenty brains were normal, but 56 showed macroscopic abnormalities with definite deviations of the sulcogyral pattern in the temporal lobes. They noted that the sulcogyral pattern of the lower temporal regions in humans appeared between the seventh and eighth foetal month, while the parahippocampal gyrus and entorhinal region is formed at an earlier stage approximately the sixth foetal month. They discussed a genetically-induced disturbed migration in the entorhinal region towards the end of the fifth month, which may be responsible for these findings.

Many of the temporal lobe changes reported, for example, by Bogerts et al. and Scheibel et al. were in the left hemisphere, but in their studies this was the only one examined. In the investigation of Jeste and Lohr (1989), maximum findings were in the left hemisphere, and this has been supported by other data. Brown et al. (1986) compared the brains of patients meeting the strict criteria for affective disorder and schizophrenia, and noted that the latter had larger temporal horns of the lateral ventricle and thinner parahippocampal gyri. The greatest differences were noted in the left hemisphere. Crow and colleagues (1989) compared brains of patients with schizophrenia, to those suffering from Alzheimer type dementia and to controls. They noted ventricular enlargement, especially of the posterior and temporal horn of the lateral ventricle, in comparison to controls and patients with Alzheimer type dementia. The abnormality was highly selective for the left hemisphere. They speculated that one mechanism of the temporal horn enlargement could be arrest of cerebral growth since the size of the temporal horn decreases during development. This arrest could be related to exogenous or endogenous factors, although their own work favours the interpretation that it is related to genetic mechanisms.

These pathological studies, summarised in Table 11.1, are supported by the neurochemical data supplied by Reynolds (1983). Although most neurochemical studies in schizophrenia relate to testing the dopamine hypothesis (for review see Trimble, 1988), and several studies suggest increases in dopamine receptor density in limbic system or related areas, Reynolds (1983) assessed laterality in relationship to neurochemical findings. In a study which has now been replicated, he compared

TABLE 11.1. *Studies Showing Hippocampal or Parahippocampal Pathology in Schizophrenia*

Study	H	PH
Nieto and Escobar, 1972	*	—
Stevens, 1982	*	—
Bogerts et al., 1983, 1985	*	—
Falkai et al., 1988	—	*
Kovelman and Scheibel, 1984	*	—
Jeste and Lohr, 1989	*	—
Jakob and Beckmann, 1989	—	*
Brown et al., 1986	—	*

*pathology noted
(H) hippocampus, (PH) parahippocampal gyrus, (—) not examined

brains from patients with schizophrenia to controls and noted that dopamine was increased in the amygdala of the schizophrenic patients selectively on the left side.

One other neurochemical study of interest that relates to temporal lobe dysfunction in schizophrenia is that of Ferrier et al. (1984). They reported cholecystokinin to be reduced in the temporal cortex, especially in the hippocampus and amygdala of patients with negative symptoms; somatostatin was decreased in the hippocampus; while vasoactive-intestinal peptide (VIP) was increased in the amygdala of those with positive symptoms.

EEG STUDIES

These neurochemical and neuropathological studies are supported by EEG and radiological data. Soon after the introduction of the EEG into clinical practice, reports of abnormalities in schizophrenia appeared (Hill, 1950). These were largely of paroxysmal and nonparoxysmal dysrhythmias, sometimes with features similar to those seen in the EEGs of patients with epilepsy. Temporal lobe abnormalities in schizophrenia have been reported frequently, with a tendency to be greater on the left (Abrahams and Taylor, 1979).

Using intracerebral implanted electrodes, Heath (1982) investigated 63 patients with psychosis, 38 of whom were diagnosed as having schizophrenia. Spiking was seen in the septal region which includes the septal nuclei, the nucleus accumbens, the olfactory tubercle and the diagonal band, as well as parts of the gyrus rectus. As noted in Chapter 4, this area has extensive frontal and temporal connections.

Heath noted changes in the septal area when patients were actively psychotic, and in many cases the EEG abnormalities were not observed on surface recordings. Neither were similar findings seen in chronic pain control patients. Violence and aggression were associated with hippocampal and amygdala discharges. Similar findings, especially with regard to the septal region, have been reported by others (Rickles, 1969; Sem-Jacobsen et al., 1956).

Using telemetred EEG during psychotic behaviour in schizophrenic patients, Stevens and Livermore (1978) identified so-called ramp patterns, characterised by a monotonic decline in power from lowest to highest frequencies, which can also be seen in epileptic patients during subcortical spike activity. These were seen only in schizophrenic patients and not in controls, and 50% of paranoid patients with auditory hallucinations had left-sided ramps with increased slow activity. Psychotic events recorded clinically were associated with suppression of left temporal alpha frequencies.

RADIOLOGICAL STUDIES

Much of the CT literature in schizophrenia (for review see Trimble, 1988) has to do with ventricular enlargement, especially of the lateral, third, and fourth ventricles. These are well-replicated findings in investigations on groups of patients with schizophrenia. A number of studies have specifically looked at temporal lobe structures, although these are poorly visualised by CT, and it is the more recent studies with MRI which have revealed most differences. McCarley et al. (1989) compared the size of CSF spaces in schizophrenic patients and compared them with controls. Overall, 10 of the 18 CT measures were significantly enlarged in the schizophrenic group. These abnormalities were then correlated with electrophysiological findings and clinical measurements. Left sylvian fissure enlargement was highly correlated with a left temporal scalp region feature of the auditory P300 that differentiated schizophrenic patients from controls, and both the enlargement and the P300 were significantly correlated with positive symptoms.

Four investigations have specifically examined temporal lobe structure in schizophrenia with MRI. Besson et al. (1987) noted no significant differences in T1 values between schizophrenic patients and controls, but reported that patients with high positive symptom scores showed increased values in left medial temporal structures, compared with those with low scores. Suddath et al. (1989) compared grey and white matter volumes in the temporal lobes of schizophrenia and controls and found that the volume of temporal lobe grey matter was 20% smaller in the patients. Anatomically, the areas corresponded to those areas of the temporal lobe containing the amygdala and anterior hippocampus, and the right temporal lobe was significantly larger than the left, although this data was obtained for the controls as well.

Johnstone et al. (1989) used MRI to assess temporal lobe structure in schizophrenics, patients with bipolar affective disorder, and normal controls. Compared with the nonschizophrenic groups, the patients with schizophrenia had a significantly smaller left temporal area.

Suddath et al. (1989) examined 15 pairs of monozygotic twins discordant for schizophrenia. Quantitative analysis of T1-weighted values at the level of the pes hippocampi showed the hippocampus to be smaller on the left in 14 affected twins compared with their control sibling, and smaller on the right in 13. Overall, left-sided changes predominated.

Another imaging technique that has been brought to this issue is that of positron emission tomography (PET). As with structural imaging techniques, virtually all studies that have been undertaken have shown differences between controls and schizophrenic patients, much emphasis having been placed in earlier studies on hypofrontality and changes of basal ganglia metabolism (for review see Trimble, 1988). With regard to laterality and temporal lobe findings, Gur et al. (1985), in unmedicated patients, showed higher resting left hemisphere cerebral blood flow, and when patients undertook a spatial task, decreases of anterior left hemisphere activity were noted compared with controls. De Lisi and colleagues (1989), using 2-deoxy-glucose, compared metabolic rate in the temporal lobes in 21 medication-free patients and matched controls. The schizophrenics had significantly increased mean and maximum metabolic rates in both temporal lobes, compared with controls, but the schizophrenics had significantly higher glucose use in the left when compared with the right temporal lobe. Using region of interest analysis, this difference was present along all structures measured, being least marked for the superior temporal area, and increasing inferiorly (superior hippocampus, midtemporal, inferior hippocampus, inferior temporal). Significant correlations between a psychopathology rating scale (the BPRS) and the superior temporal gyrus left/right ratio were noted for suspiciousness, thought disorder, disorganised speech, hallucinations and emotional withdrawal.

Finally, Wiesel and colleagues (1987), using C11 glucose as a tracer, examined different brain regions in healthy male volunteers and 20 drug-free schizophrenic patients. With regard to temporal lobe findings, left/right asymmetry was noted in the temporal lobe (in area 22), the metabolic rates of the schizophrenic patients being lower on the left compared to controls. Whether the different direction of this compared with other studies was related to tracer or to patient selection is unclear. In this study, analysis of amygdala findings revealed differences between hebephrenics and paranoid patients, the latter having higher metabolic rates in the left amygdala.

These PET findings should be taken in conjuction with the findings in psychosis and epilepsy reported by Trimble and colleagues (Gallhofer et al., 1985), where hypometabolic areas were found in association with temporal lobe epilepsy, but maximum in the left hemisphere in psychotic patients.

These studies of schizophrenic patients lead to the following conclusions. Schizophrenia is a neurological illness with the maximum pathology affecting limbic system structures (for review see Trimble, 1988). The above review relates mainly to findings in temporal lobe structures, which have been noted to be abnormal using neuropathological, EEG, and radiological techniques. Table 11.1 lists nine studies which have shown hippocampal pathology in schizophrenia, and it is difficult not to conclude that this structure is intimately related to its pathogenesis. Associations with certain symptoms have been suggested by certain authors; in particular, positive symptoms (Stevens, 1986; Besson et al., 1987), hallucinations, speech disturbance, suspiciousness, and hostility (De Lisi, 1989; McCarley, 1989). Although not universally found, a tendency to maximum dysfunction in the left hemisphere has been reported, although there are some negative findings. This is remarkable in view of the data presented in Chapter 9 and reviewed in Tables 9.3 and 9.4. The conclusion that the schizophrenia-like psychoses of epilepsy and schizophrenia have common underlying areas of anatomical dysfunction within the limbic system seems secure. It is difficult not to conclude that patients with schizophrenia, particularly those with positive symptoms, are likely to show limbic system disturbances if looked for; the hippocampus, amygdala, and parahippocampal gyrus, especially on the left side, are most likely to be involved. Finally, it is relevant to the issue of the links between epilepsy and psychopathology that the most common form of epilepsy involved is that related to temporal lobe abnormalities, and that the lesions of this form of seizure disorder are often found in the hippocampus and amygdala.

THE SCHIZOPHRENIA-LIKE PSYCHOSES OF EPILEPSY

There have been several explanations for the pathogenesis of these psychoses. The first issue relates to whether or not they truly resemble schizophrenia in the absence of epilepsy. Early conclusions were reached by several authors. Gibbs et al. (1938) believed that the relationship between epilepsy and schizophrenia was a positive one and that there were few differences between the presentations of psychiatric disorders in patients with and those without epilepsy. Hoch (1943) thought in some patients it was "clinically impossible to differentiate the epileptic psychosis from schizophrenia" while in others, certain symptoms indicated an organic psychosis. Slater and Beard (1963b) used the term *schizophrenia-like* to emphasise the similarity of the phenomenology, but stressed differences; notably, the way that epileptic patients with psychosis tended to remain friendlier and more cooperative and to retain affective warmth when compared with schizophrenics without epilepsy. They also noted the relative infrequency of catatonic symptoms.

Phenomenological comparisons and similarities were also noted in the PSE studies of Perez et al. (1985) and Toone et al. (1982a). The latter also emphasised the underrepresentation of catatonic features.

Bruens (1971) denied that the psychoses of epilepsy could be brought under the heading of any classic psychiatric syndrome, stating that none of his cases fulfilled strict criteria for the diagnosis of schizophrenia as laid out by some German authors. He noted there was "no praecox feeling."

The suggestion which emerges, therefore, is that these psychoses differ from process schizophrenia in certain fundamental ways from a phenomenological viewpoint; in particular, with the maintenance of affective warmth and lack of hebephrenic deterioration with personality dilapidation (see also Table 3.7). It would seem appropriate, therefore, to refer to them as schizophrenia-like psychoses of epilepsy. Such nosological specificity also applies to some of the more extreme personality changes that have been outlined (see Chapter 8), notably, the Geschwind syndrome.

With regard to the pathogenesis, various theories have been suggested. A genetic relationship was ruled by Hoch (1943), who noted no increase of schizophrenia in the consanguinity of epileptic patients, and vice versa. Likewise, in the family studies of Slater, there was no specific predisposition to schizophrenia in the schizophrenia-like psychoses of epilepsy, and Slater regarded the latter as "non-endogenous but symptomatic," which could be regarded as "a phenocopy of a genetically determined condition" (p. 149). The only study to suggest a significant hereditary component was that of Jensen and Larsen (1979b) on a highly selected group of patients who had temporal lobe surgery. The relatives were not personally interviewed, and the psychiatric diagnosis of the relatives is not given.

Several early authors stressed psychological interpretations (Ziehen, 1902). Pond (1957) felt that the continuing disruption created by recurrent ictal and postictal alterations of the mental state, especially as seen in temporal lobe epilepsy, may be influential for the later development of psychosis. This view receives only minimal support from the studies that have investigated the relationship between auras and psychosis, in the sense that the association with psychopathology relates to a limbic system origin of the aura rather than content (see Chapter 6), and the only study to specifically study content (Taylor and Lochery, 1987) did not find a relationship.

Bruens (1971) emphasised both organic (temporal lobe) and psychodynamic factors, noting with regard to the latter the disturbed overprotective environment in which epileptic patients live. He felt that organic and psychodynamic factors "potentiate" each other. Ramani and Gumnit (1982) felt that the psychoses were "the reaction of a constitutionally predisposed individual to the continual physiological or psychological impact of recurrent seizures." Other authors who have emphasised sociological factors include Wolf (1988), patients in his investigations who became psychotic being vocationally and socially disintegrated with little or no professional training. Social integration was seen as a stabilising factor in a potentially psychotogenic situation. Likewise, social factors were considered important by Ferguson and Rayport (1965).

The problems with these theories is that they fail to explain the observed associations between psychoses of epilepsy and seizure expression, the link with limbic seizures, and the laterality effects.

Several authors have drawn attention to common factors shared by epilepsy, the schizophrenia-like psychoses of epilepsy, and schizophrenia (Table 11.2).

One of the earliest recorded abnormalities was that of temporal lobe pathology,

TABLE 11.2. *Some Links Between Epilepsy, Schizophrenia-like Psychoses of Epilepsy, and Schizophrenia*

Pathology:	MTS and/or disorganisation of temporal, specifically hippocampal structures. Subcortical, basal forebrain and cerebellar findings.
EEG:	Paroxysmal and "epileptiform" discharges. Depth spikes and rhythmical discharges, especially in amygdala, hippocampus, and basal forebrain.
CT/MRI:	Increased ventricular size: temporal lobe changes.
PET:	Hypo- or hypermetabolism of temporal structures, hypofrontality.

initially outlined by Bouchet and Cazauvieilh (1825). This issue was tackled again recently by Stevens (1986). She reported on the neuropathological and clinical findings of six cases of epilepsy followed by psychosis. Four demonstrated significant left hippocampal sclerosis, but for these cases the right hemisphere was not available for examination. Gliosis and mild degenerative changes were also noted in the pallidum, brainstem, tegmentum, periaqueductal or periventricular regions of the basal forebrain, and the thalamus. Stevens described these changes as "similar to changes observed in our larger series of patients with schizophrenia" (p. 133). Stevens concluded that: "The association of the MTS and severe behaviour disturbances . . . is related . . . to a combination of MTS plus pathology in subcortical, limbic, pallidal, thalamic, hypothalamic and periventricular regions" (p. 133).

However, MTS was not seen as crucial in the sense that the interictal paranoid hallucinatory psychoses occurred in some patients without MTS. It should be noted that MTS is not exclusive to epilepsy, being reported in nine out of 28 schizophrenic patients without epilepsy in the series of Stevens, although unassociated with conspicuous pyramidal cell loss which is seen in cases of epilepsy and psychosis. Stevens favoured scattered lesions in a number of subcortical areas which receive projections from medial temporolimbic structures as responsible for interictal psychopathology.

EEG similarities have been noted since the earliest of the EEG investigations (Gibbs et al., 1936; Jasper et al., 1939). They noted how pathological dysrhythmias were seen in epilepsy, but also in schizophrenia. Gibbs et al. (1936) wrote: "The disorders of behaviour encountered in individuals who display . . . schizophrenic . . . traits, when accompanied by the disorders of cortical rhythm present in epilepsy, suggest that all these might be considered various manifestations of epilepsy" (p. 266). These authors criticised too rigid a terminology, and suggested that physicians should seek freedom of thought, making terminology secondary to underlying "vital processes."

Jasper et al. (1939) noted: "We could detect no single specific form of activity in the electroencephalograms from patients diagnosed schizophrenic which would distinguish them, as a group, from those classified as epileptic or as normal" (p. 839). "Epileptiform activity" was noted in 21% of schizophrenics, and in 6% of normals.

These cortical studies were complemented by the elegant studies of Heath (1962) with implanted electrodes. He drew distinctions between the depth recordings of seizure patients and those with schizophrenia. However, the anatomical regions from which the abnormal recordings were obtained were the same in both groups, although seizure patients had more pronounced abnormalities in the hippocampus and amygdala and less in the septal region, while the schizophrenic and other psychotic patients had abnormalities predominantly in the septal region. Epileptic patients, when they become psychotic, showed septal abnormalities. For Heath it was the involvement of similar anatomical structures which lead to the development of psychotic behaviour.

The interictal EEG similarities in limbic areas in epilepsy and schizophrenia were underlined by the paper of Kendrick and Gibbs (1957). They studied 75 patients who had been psychotic for a prolonged period of time; 13 had psychomotor epilepsy and 62 had psychosis without epilepsy. Depth electrodes were implanted in a variety of areas, and waking and sleeping recordings taken. Figure 11.1, taken from their paper, shows their results. Spiking was detected in medial temporal and frontal structures in 13 patients with psychomotor epilepsy and psychosis and in 62 patients with psychosis and no epilepsy. The authors commented that almost 50% of schizophrenic cases had a clearly defined spike-focus in the anterior temporal region and/ or in the frontal areas. The medial temporal lobe was thus frequently involved.

Other similarities between schizophrenia and the schizophrenia-like psychoses of epilepsy include CT changes, notably, ventricular size (Perez et al., 1985), MRI evidence of disturbed limbic system structure (see above), and changes of function in studies using positron emission tomography. These do not abate with temporal lobectomy, attesting to their continuing presence and significance interictally (Radtke et al., 1989).

MECHANISMS

In view of these findings, most authors start their explanations of association between epilepsy and psychosis with observations of links between psychoses and temporal lobe epilepsy (Chapters 8 and 9), noting the extensive literature which emphasises the intimate association between the temporal lobes and modulation of behaviour and emotion (Chapter 4).

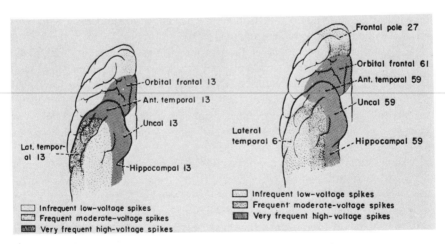

FIG. 11.1. Sites of spiking in limbic structures in patients with psychosis and epilepsy (left) and psychosis without epilepsy (right). Intensity of spiking is indicated by stippling and crosshatching. (Kendrick and Gibbs, 1957)

Berrios (Chapter 1) discussed the options prevailing a century ago, and Slater and Beard (1963a,b) returned to some of these. Their arguments would reject 1a and 1b, and emphasise 2c, and variants of 2aii (see page 12). Thus, either epilepsy was a precipitating factor for the schizophrenia-like illness, or the schizophrenia-like illness was epileptic in origin. They dismissed the first explanation on the grounds that epileptic psychotic patients lack prepsychotic personalities of the schizoid type and, if anything, note differing personality traits including viscosity, aggression, religiosity, and egocentricity in association with the psychoses. They also pointed out, on the basis of a follow-up study, that in contrast to the expected deterioration with schizophrenia, the schizophrenia-like psychoses tend to leave the personality substantially undamaged. Thus, on their follow-up of 93% of their patients, 16% had ceased having seizures, and the schizophrenia-like symptoms had resolved or improved in 68%.

Slater and Beard pointed to the predominance of temporal lobe abnormalities and the clinical phenomenology. They then discussed the aetiological relationships that could exist between the epilepsy and the psychoses, either seizures themselves being the adequate cause, or there being a basic disorder of function manifesting itself both as seizures and as psychosis. Their data supported the second hypothesis; namely, that underlying the epilepsy was some process which at one stage was liable to lead to seizures, and at another to the psychoses. The process they suggested was an organic lesion in the temporal lobes, pointing in their series to the high frequency of a history of head injuries, the evidence of organic personality change, and the air encephalography changes. They acknowledged that patients rated by them as hebephrenic may be aetiologically different. The necessity to distinguish between phenomenological types emerges in some other studies, notably, in that of Perez and Trimble (1980), where epileptic patients rated as nuclear schizophrenic clearly have a number of distinguishing features in comparison with those classified with other forms of schizophrenia.

The view that the emergence of the psychoses is associated with identifiable structural brain damage was also supported by the studies of Kristensen and Sindrup (1978a,b), the pathological studies of the temporal lobectomy series by Taylor (1975) and by Jensen and Larsen (1979b) and Bruton (1988). However, evidence for links to a specific pathology, either hamartomas or specific gangliogliomas, cannot be held up: patients with MTS also develop psychoses (Jensen and Larsen, 1979b; Sherwin et al., 1982; Bruton, 1988).

The suggestion that seizures are more relevant than underlying structural lesions emerges from several sources. Flor-Henry (1969) emphasised links between seizures and psychosis (as had earlier been shown by Landolt) and links between psychosis and infrequent expression of seizures in his series. He criticised the data of Slater and Beard (1963) on the grounds that there were no controls, and he emphasised that in his own controlled study the incidence of identifiable organic abnormalities was the same in psychotic and nonpsychotic epileptic patients. Flor-Henry concludes: "Epileptic psychoses are not 'organic' psychoses, in the general non-specific sense of the term but are truly 'epileptic' psychoses fundamentally related to epilepsy rather than to associated brain damage" (p. 389).

He reflected that underlying patterns of abnormal neuronal activity, especially in the dominant temporal lobes, were fundamentally responsible for the schizophrenic syndrome. In contrast, manic-depressive psychoses associated with temporal lobe epilepsy were related to infrequently manifested generalised seizures, hinting that neuronal systems responsible for generalised seizures were more critical in determining the appearance of the manic-depressive states. The link here to the biological antagonism of ECT is obvious.

Symonds (1962), in a discussion of Slater's findings, noted that damage to the temporal lobes occurred in other neurological conditions, but usually did not cause a schizophrenia-like condition. He then referred to the "epileptogenic disorder of function." He acknowledged that abnormalities of function continued interictally, and said "this background disorder may cause symptoms other than seizures" (p. 4). The continuing interictal abnormality of function has now been noted in many studies, including depth electrode studies and more recently the metabolic PET data. Symonds (1962) further continued: "It is not loss of neurones in the temporal lobe that is responsible for the psychosis, but the disorderly activity of those that remain, and that this disorderly activity is of the kind that is also likely to cause seizures" (p. 5).

These ideas have much more to do with the continuing process of epilepsy, and clearly make the distinction between epilepsy viewed purely as a disorder of seizures and epilepsy viewed as a disorder or cerebral function of which seizures are but one manifestation. A similar theme was taken up by Taylor (1975) where he discussed abnormal cerebral organization, especially referring to areas outside the immediate temporal focus.

The radiological evidence, particularly CT, MRI and PET has emphasised that structural lesions do not underlie the psychoses but may influence the pattern of symptoms, while disturbance of function interictally is not only extensive in psychotic patients, but it also affects areas outside the immediate anterior temporal lobes. Studies with MRI (Conlon et al., 1988) reveal fairly well-circumscribed structural changes in the anterior temporal lobe in patients with temporal lobe epilepsy, but the metabolic changes are more widespread, affecting temporal, basal ganglia, and frontal regions (Gallhofer et al., 1985). These data touch on underlying anatomical connections between the medial temporal structures, maximally affected in temporal lobe epilepsy and other areas of the limbic system, embraced by the concept of the extended amygdala (see page 43). The direct links between the anterior temporal lobes and the basal forebrain and frontal cortex reveal that the influence of damage to circumscribed areas of the temporal lobe may be wide. These ideas emphasise the value of identifying patients who suffer from limbic epilepsy and distinctions between the different forms of temporal lobe epilepsy. The data are reinforced by the medial temporal site of origin of pathology in psychotic patients who come to surgery (Bruton, 1988).

One issue which has created considerable discussion has been the finding of Slater and Beard (1963a) of a fairly constant relationship between the age of onset of epilepsy and the age of onset of psychosis, reviewed in Chapter 9. Stevens suggested that this relationship is an artefact based on the number of patients with anterior temporal lobe spikes on the EEG rising with age in a manner which correlates with the age-related incidence of presentations with psychosis. Toone (1981) does not accept this explanation, noting that the age of onset for temporal lobe epilepsy peaks between 25 and 50 years, whereas the first admission for schizophrenia lies between 20 and 40 years for the majority of patients. The peak for psychomotor seizures in the series given by Gibbs and Gibbs (1952) seems to be between 15 and 30 years.

An important aetiological link between seizures and psychosis is suggested by the laterality findings, especially that between the left hemisphere and the schizophrenia-like psychoses. Again, this has been criticised on the grounds that patients with epilepsy tend to have an increased frequency of left-sided pathology without psychoses, especially if selected populations such as hospital referral patients are examined. These criticisms cannot explain the more circumscribed association between specific forms of psychoses, especially schizophrenia-like psychoses with first rank symptoms of Schneider (nuclear schizophrenia) and the left hemisphere, as has emerged from studies of phenomenology. Further, they must counter the increased number of findings which now clearly emphasise a laterality effect with a predominance of left-sided abnormalities in patients with schizophrenia who do not have epilepsy (reviewed above). Finally, the laterality of the focus in epileptic populations without psychoses are variable, depending on the series. For example, in the extensive series of Juul-Jensen (1964), where laterality could be established, it was left-sided in 52%. In the series of Gibbs and Gibbs (1952) the focus of psychomotor seizures was left in 35%, right in 36% and bilateral in 29%. Curie et al. (1971) give a figure of 60% left and 40% right.

Explanations for the development of the schizophrenia-like psychoses in epilepsy, therefore, need to take into account the age of onset of epilepsy, the site of the underlying pathology, the length of time between the onset of epilepsy and the onset of the psychosis, and maximum disturbance of function in the dominant hemisphere. Tentative explanations have been given. Several authors (Taylor, 1975; Perez et al., 1985) have postulated that the disorganised left hemisphere leads to a susceptibility to abnormalities of symbolic language, especially if the disturbance is present during the time of language development and when emotional bonding to peers and parents is paramount. Taylor (1977) puts it succinctly: "Supposing there were, in the developing brain, a lesion which provoked epilepsy but which was not gross enough to produce a major reorganization of developmental strategy in the brain. Such a lesion would, in youth, not necessarily produce serious consequences while the language system was extensively deployed through the hemisphere, though it may create some diffusion of language organization. As the normal contraction and condensation of language proceeds, however, the disruption created by the lesion may increase quite markedly and suddenly" (p. 36). Or, as he also said

(Taylor, 1975): "It is scarcely surprising that schizophrenic symptoms should exist in the presence of dysfunction, throughout early development, in those territories critical for speech and integration" (p. 253).

There is, indeed, evidence that patients with temporal lobe epilepsy show language disturbances (Hermann and Wyler, 1988) and that some of the memory deficits associated with epilepsy may represent anomic problems (Mayeux et al., 1980).

Trimble and colleagues (Perez et al., 1985) specifically suggest an association between schizophrenia-like disturbance and temporal lobe epilepsy, raising the issue as to whether this model for schizophrenia with positive symptoms differs from process schizophrenia in the absence of epilepsy by not having associated frontal lobe pathology. There is absence of symptoms and signs associated with frontal lobe dysfunction, as seen in more chronic forms of schizophrenia with personality deterioration. Frontal lobe function in patients with epilepsy has been poorly investigated, but in schizophrenia, in the absence of epilepsy, there is now considerable evidence from neuropathological, EEG, neuropsychological, and radiological, structural, and functional studies that the frontal lobes are involved, at least in a significant percentage of patients (for review see Trimble, 1988).

The observation that psychoses develop after temporal lobectomy (see Chapter 7) is further support for the idea that the cerebral disorganization underlying the psychoses is not totally related to the anterior temporal limbic area, but must represent more widespread dysfunction. Two mechanisms that have been suggested relate to alterations of amine metabolism and kindling.

Lamprecht (1973) and Trimble (1977) have emphasised the antithetical relationship between dopamine and schizophrenia, dopamine agonism tending to be psychotogenic but also having anticonvulsant properties, dopamine antagonism provoking seizures but being antipsychotic. This mechanism, discussed in relationship to forced normalisation in Chapter 5, may also play a role in chronically developing psychoses, gradually increasing dopamine activity explaining the disappearance of seizures in some patients. The only data that relate to this are those of Peters (1979), who noted low CSF HVA which might suggest upregulation of postsynaptic receptors, and the recent PET study of Sherwin and colleagues (Dyve et al., 1989). The latter investigation quantitatively assessed dopa decarboxylase activity in epileptic patients with a left unilateral mesial temporal epileptic focus using radioactively labelled fluoro-dopa. The amygdala and hippocampus showed significant increases in dopa decarboxylase activity, suggesting enhanced dopamine turnover.

Kindling, while being an experimental model for epilepsy, may have clinical relevance beyond epilepsy (Bolwig and Trimble, 1989). Kindling is most easily elicited from mediotemporal limbic structures, for example, the amygdala, but when forebrain areas are experimentally kindled, particularly catecholaminergic regions, disturbances of behaviour rather than seizures are elicited (Stevens and Livermore, 1978). There is experimental animal data showing that following kindling of the amygdala, mesolimbic dopaminergic sensitivity increases, and there are increased D-2 receptor densities in the nucleus accumbens (Csernansky et al., 1988). The suggestion is that ongoing subictal activity in mesial temporal structures may thus kindle downstream limbic nuclei, altering their neuromodulator function and, with regard to dopamine, increasing activity and hence the liability to psychosis. This further fits with the underlying anatomical concept of the extended amygdala and the anatomical connections outlined in Chapter 4. It is difficult to ignore the growing literature on the neurochemistry of schizophrenia in which the same do-pamine-rich limbic forebrain areas are thought to be related, at least in part, to the development of the psychoses (for review see Trimble, 1988).

The evidence that kindling is an important mechanism for the development of the psychoses of epilepsy is, however, conjectural. Although there are cases of kindling recognised in humans (for review see Bolwig and Trimble, 1989), they are rare. The main argument against kindling relates to the follow-up studies of patients with epilepsy and psychosis. Glithero and Slater (1963) commented that "the excellent epileptic result was accompanied by a favourable development in the psychosis." In another recent follow-up study, Kenwood and Betts (1988) presented data on a group of hospitalised psychotic epileptic patients followed up for 20 years. Again, there was a relationship between improvement of seizures and a diminution of the psychoses. In contrast, Feinstein and Ron (1990) followed up 65 psychotic patients with unequivocal evidence of brain pathology, 37 of whom suffered from seizures. Patients with epilepsy were more likely to have psychotic relapses and to receive psychiatric care than those without epilepsy, and the occurrence of the psychotic relapse did not seem to be related to the extent of the seizure control.

Positive and Negative Symptoms

Hughlings Jackson (1875) elegantly discussed the relationship between cerebral lesions and symptoms. His introduction of the terms *positive and negative symptoms* has recently been revived in neuropsychiatry, although often without an understanding of the mechanism behind his theory (Trimble, 1986). Although Hughlings Jackson explicitly adopted psychophysical parallelism in his understanding of mind-brain interactions, in explaining his concept of positive and negative symptoms, he frequently discussed "mental" changes. Before integrating some of his ideas into an understanding of the epileptic psychoses, it is germane to return to the writing of Jaspers. It was noted in Chapter 3 how Jaspers developed a descriptive psycho-pathology and made certain fundamental distinctions, notably, between understanding and explanation, or what is meaningful and what is causal. Essentially, causal connections are directly related to the somatic realm and are deduced by the methods of the natural sciences. However, phenomenology demands both explanation and understanding and draws a distinction between form and content. The interpretations of epileptic psychoses have been variously those which depend upon understanding (people who have sudden repeated loss of consciousness and thus are in danger, who are unable to get an occupation, and who are unpopular amongst their peers will become paranoid) and explanation (disturbance in the temporal lobes at a certain point in life leads to the development of phenomena which are beyond the nature of meaningful connections). The latter changes may be seen as a consequence of process rather than development, the process being linked with that which, at various times, provokes epileptic seizures.

Jaspers himself was pessimistic about neurological localisation in relationship to psychic entities, and while Hughlings Jackson ostensibly took the same position, he actually wrote a considerable amount concerning "mental" activity and its relationship to brain disorder. He did not believe in the strict concept of cerebral localisation, and his theories of brain action depended on several features, especially positive and negative phenomena and the concept of dissolution. Destruction of tissue would result in negative symptoms, but release of subjacent activity of other healthy areas of the brain would lead to positive symptoms. He noted that in all cases of insanity the principle of dissolution, the level of evolution that remains, and the positive and negative symptoms needed to be considered.

In discussing postepileptic mania he referred to the negative and positive element. The negative element is related to loss of consciousness, while dissolution leaves the activity of other "nervous arrangements" to "spring into activity," and hence the development of the mania. Although this model applied to ictal events, (Jackson 1880, 1881) he also applied it to cases of insanity in other settings. For example: "Illusions, delusions, extravagant conduct, and abnormal emotional states in an insane person signify evolution, not dissolution; they signify evolution going on in what remains intact of the mutilated highest centres—in what disease, effecting so much dissolution, has spared" (Jackson, 1894). The negative mental state could be slight, while the positive one elaborate.

With regard to epileptic psychosis, it is possible to unite the biological and phenomenological by acknowledging the presence of a disrupting focus in one or another of the temporal lobes, particularly during crucial phases of development. This leads to the development of negative symptoms, perhaps in the form of memory deficits or loss of insight, but also to positive symptoms, ultimately with delusions and hallucinations. The latter for their presence are dependent upon cortical and subcortical areas removed from the site of the abnormal focus. The concept of reaction here is also important. Thus, the reactions of the brain to various exogenous insults and endogenous aberrations, which might include a pathological lesion that may lead to a seizure, will lead to a skewing of the relationship of other areas of brain to the focus of change, and ultimately towards their function in relationship to environmental events. Such reaction will differ from individual to individual, again reflected by Jackson, who, in his four factors in insanities (Jackson, 1894), discussed not only the different depths and rates of dissolution, but also "different persons who have undergone that dissolution . . . different local bodily states and different external circumstances of the persons who have undergone that dissolution" (p. 615).

Stevens (1988) had developed a biochemical variant of this view, hinted at earlier by Landolt's concepts of the development of forced normalisation (p. 69), suggesting increased reactivity of some parts of the brain to focal areas of dysfunction. She notes that "microseizures" not uncommonly arise within the brain during normal brain function, and in order to prevent spread of these microseizures, inhibitory circuits must have developed in surrounding areas. These would involve inhibitory neurotransmitters such as GABA, dopamine, and noradrenaline. Increased inhibition of physiological microseizures, indeed, the development of microseizures at times or in situations when they are not physiologically required, could lead to an enhanced inhibitory surround or "reaction" in limbic areas, such reaction being related to the development of the psychosis.

Stimulation of limbic system structures, notably the hippocampus and amygdala, lead to experiential phenomena (Gloor et al., 1982), essentially positive phenomena. Gloor (1991), based on data obtained from stimulation studies, noted that it is illogical to assume that reproduction of experiences known to be dependent on the anatomical and functional integrity of medial temporal structures should arise as a consequence of their inactivation. He suggested that experiential phenomena are positive expressions of the activity of neurones involved in or affected by epileptic discharges. He based his arguments on the concept of a distributive matrix of excitation and inhibition which relates to the neuronal representation of experiences and how activation at one point within a network can re-create a whole pattern. Thus, limited discharge in a group of neurones in medial temporal structures may lead to the re-creation of experiences dependent on widely distributed matrixes. In the setting of a seizure, when neuronal activity becomes very disturbed, loss of consciousness will occur, and the positive phenomena will be obliterated. Using this model, however, it is possible to see how recurrent abnormal function in these structures, which may possibly be recorded interictally as abnormal electrical activity when electrodes are in the right place, could also lead to similar phenomena with a "kindling" of long-lasting emotional and behavioural changes. The emphasis here is on the development of symptoms or possible syndromes and not of disease. In this context, the development of chronic interictal psychoses following bouts of paroxysmal peri-ictal psychoses, seen and recorded in several patients (see Chapter 6), must be relevant.

The results suggesting that first rank symptoms may be specially linked to temporal limbic dysfunction are of interest. Thus, Schneider himself referred to first rank symptoms as "grouped together under the concept of permeability of the barrier between the individual and his environment." Anatomically the medial temporal structures, especially the hippocampus and parahippocampal gyrus, may be seen as correlates providing such permeability.

Using such models as the developmental models of Taylor (1975), the development of the schizophrenia-like psychoses of epilepsy, with their dependence mainly on the left side of the brain, become more plausible. Possibly similar mechanisms may relate to affective disturbances and the right temporal lobe, although findings in this area are far more restricted, and theoretical mechanisms less clearly developed. Further, non-NS seems to have differing associations compared with NS, emphasising the importance of precision when defining clinical pictures and not the assumption that all psychoses fall under the same umbrella.

An important issue is why do only a certain percentage of patients with temporal lobe discharges develop psychoses? A possible explanation rests with the pathological data. Scheibel (1991) has drawn attention to the similarities of both schizophrenia and temporal lobe epilepsy, especially from pathological studies. He noted that in both syndromes the hippocampus is the main site of structural change, with loss of neurones in MTS and disarray of pyramidal cells in the hippocampus of brains from schizophrenics. He concludes, in comparing temporal lobe epilepsy and schizophrenia, that "the schizophrenic syndrome is considered here, not necessarily as a closely-related disease process but rather as an example of another, long-term, incapacitating syndrome apparently related to limbic lobe dysfunction" (p. 73).

Thus, in schizophrenia the most prominent changes are pyramidal cell disarray at interface zones, prosubiculum and CA1, CA1 and CA2, and CA4 regions. The pathology of temporal lobe epilepsy itself is so variable (see Chapter 4). Lesions such as hamartomas occur more frequently in the amygdala, while in MTS it is the CA1 region of the hippocampus that is most involved. If the study of Jeste and Lohr is replicated and the major changes in schizophrenia are found in CA3 and CA4, and CA1 is relatively unaffected, then it may be that patients with temporal lobe epilepsy with sparing of the Sommer sector and dentate gyrus but who have cell loss and gliosis or some other pathological change in the end folium will be the patients with maximum vulnerability. It seems to be the case that the CA3 area is a meeting point for much sensory information while the function of CA1 is as yet largely unknown.

The predominant links of CA3 and CA4 are to the septum and the opposite hippocampus, while CA1 and CA2 have different afferent and efferent connections. The role of the septum in psychotic states has been discussed above. Further, the fact that in experimental models of epilepsy, spikes arise in CA3 suggests further neurophysiological links between epilepsy, sites of pathology, and psychosis. In this context, it is of interest that a distinguishing feature of patients with end folium pathology in the series of Margerison and Corsellis (1966) was age of onset of seizures, similar to that in psychotic groups (see Table 9.2). However, in the study of Dam (1980) there was no association between the site of pathology in patients with epilepsy and the presence of psychosis, in spite of CA4 being the area maximally affected by MTS.

Finally, the more obvious involvement of the parahippocampal gyrus in studies of schizophrenia suggests another possible difference that may underlie the pathology of the two syndromes.

In summary, attempts to understand the development of epileptic psychosis, particularly the schizophrenia-like psychoses in epilepsy, require a willingness to go beyond direct localizationist views of neurological processes and permit some attempt to blend both psychic and somatic levels of explanation. The suggestion that temporal lobe epilepsy is a good biological model for the development of positive symptoms in neuropsychiatry has been made, and an understanding of this could be furthered through the phenomenological methodology of Jaspers and the ideas of

Hughlings Jackson. Future research on the abnormalities of function and structure of the brains of patients with epilepsy and psychoses, whether derived from neuro-pathological, electrophysiological, or radiological studies, will lead to greater understanding of the fascinating connection between the brain and the mind.

Appendix

VINCENT VAN GOGH

Vincent Willem van Gogh was born in 1853 and his illness has been, since his death by suicide in 1890, a controversial subject among biographers. The earlier view of Jaspers that van Gogh was schizophrenic appears based upon his letters and paintings rather than biographical details of his life and does not generally seem to have been supported by the artist's lack of evident deterioration between his psychotic episodes. Others have considered syphilis, alcoholism, or absinth poisoning to be likely alternatives.

Riese as well as Minkowska considered the possibility of a diagnosis of epilepsy, a view which has been most strongly propagated by French writers, most notably, Gastaut.

THE EPILEPSY OF VAN GOGH

It is known that there was a family history of epilepsy, several relatives of van Gogh being afflicted, including his mother's sister. There is substantial evidence of a seizure disorder from the physicians who actually treated him. His most famous hospitalisation was when he was at Saint-Paul-de-Mausole asylum at Saint-Remy-de-Provence. He was admitted there a few weeks following the celebrated psychotic episode in which he cut off his left ear (see below). The physician director, Dr. Peyron, stated in his report dated May 25, 1889, that there were grounds for continuing van Gogh in treatment, and wrote, "I consider . . . that M. van Gogh is subject to attacks of epilepsy." Soon after this, van Gogh was to write to his brother, Theo, that he was "epileptic probably for good." The same diagnosis was given by the intern, Dr. Felix Rey. Further, he was treated with bromides, a standard medication for epilepsy in those times.

THE PSYCHOTIC ATTACKS

The basis for the diagnosis was related to the recurrent psychotic attacks from which van Gogh suffered. On December 23, 1888, in a "state of violent excitement," he cut off a piece of his left ear and sent it as a gift to a girl called Rachel, a local prostitute. Variously interpreted as an act of symbolic castration, an inturning of his aggression towards Gauguin, a reenactment of the scene of the vanquished bull and victorious matador (van Gogh having seen bullfights in Arles), an attempt to enforce his weakening bonds with his brother, Theo, who had just become engaged; it is more likely to represent one of several confusional episodes that were well-documented in his medical history. After this episode he was found unconscious. He was admitted to hospital, but had another attack early in February after discharge. His behaviour during this one was so strange that it frightened the local people of Arles, and they brought out a public petition to have him rehospitalised. Following recovery from the latter episode, he was transferred to the asylum at Saint-Remy, and several episodes are noted in both his own correspondence and the hospital records. The attacks he had were sudden in onset but gradual in their disappearance; usually he would recover in under 2 weeks. They were heralded by disorientation, loss of concentration, and were sometimes associated with loss of consciousness. Van Gogh wrote: "I have had in all four great crises, during which I did not in the least know what I said, what I wanted, and what I did. Not taking into account that I had previously had three fainting fits without any plausible reason and without retaining the slightest remembrance of what I felt" (1888). On another occasion he wrote: "During the attacks it is terrible—then I lose consciousness of everything" (1889). In one of his episodes he ruined a Delacroix lithograph that had been sent to him by his brother. Van Gogh referred to these episodes as "grand crises" or, alternatively, "fainting spells," and it is noted that he was amnesic for them. During the attacks he had hallucinations and delusions. The hallucinations were both visual and auditory, and to him they were "real" and very frightening. He wrote of some of them in reference to his fellow patients: "During their attacks, they have also heard strange sounds and voices as I did . . . probably because the nerves of the ear are diseased and too sensitive, and in my case it was my sight as well as my hearing."

He had bizarre religious and paranoid delusions. He also reported that during these episodes people seemed to be a great distance away (micropsia), voices seemed to come from afar, and were "in reality."

At least seven attacks were specifically mentioned in his letters and in the hospital records during the time he was at Saint-Remy (a period of just over a year). It is not clear at what point in his life such episodes started, but it is known that he had suffered from episodes of dizziness for many years. These attacks were not closely interlinked with his bouts of heavy drinking.

FEATURES OF THE GESCHWIND SYNDROME

There is considerable evidence that van Gogh developed some of the features of the Geschwind syndrome noted in Chapter 8. Between attacks his intelligence remained unimpaired but he displayed hypergraphia and religiosity. The hypergraphia was evidenced not only in the classic way but also in a variant, with a prodigious output of paintings, especially in the latter years of his life. There are, thus, at least 600 letters to his brother, Theo, surviving and many others to different members of his family and other artists. In less than 2 years, while he was at Nuenen (1884–1886), he did 225 drawings, 25 water colours, and 185 oils. In Paris, between 1886 and 1888 there were about 200 oils, 10 water colours, and 40 drawings, and at Arles (1888–1890) about 185 oils, 100 drawings, and 10 water colours. These add up to approximately an oil painting every other day for at least 6 years. The repetitive nature of some of the themes of his paintings is seen when they are viewed chronologically, particularly with quasi-religious themes; for example, the olive trees.

Van Gogh came from a religious background; both his father and paternal grandfather were ministers. Religion was, therefore, a feature of his life, but religiosity became a feature of his illness. In childhood he was not known for any excessive religious zeal, and it was not until the age of 20 years that he turned increasingly to religion and spent much of his time reading the Bible. By 1886 this had become "an obsession." He considered becoming a minister and received a trial as an evangelist but was dismissed for "excessive zeal bordering on the scandalous." During this time he gave away his possessions, lived in a hovel, and became unkempt in his personal appearance.

Religious asceticism and martyrdom were a central theme in van Gogh's correspondence from 1875 to 1880. He strongly identified with Christ, taking on a portrayal of the martyred Jesus, and he read the New Testament over and over again. In 1887 he was translating the Bible into French, German, and English in four columns, with the Dutch text in addition. On Sundays, he not only went to the Dutch Reformed Church, but went on the same day to three other churches of different denominations. His religiosity fused with philosophical mysticism, and themes of suffering, death, and heaven peppered his writings. He mused on heaven and eternity, hence the paintings of the starry skies and olive trees. It is even suggested that the ear he gifted to Rachel was a religious gift with symbolic overtones. During his attacks he had delusions with religious content and said, "I have attacks such as a superstitious man might have and that I get perverted and frightful ideas about religion."

He expressed interest in the mystical, especially ghosts, and wrote on the walls of his house at Arles: "Je suis saint esprit: Je suis sain d'esprit" (I am the Holy Spirit; I am healthy of spirit).

SEXUALITY

With regard to van Gogh's sexual life, little is known. At the age of 20 years he fell in love with the engaged daughter of his London landlady, and at 29 professed love for a recently widowed cousin on his mother's side. For a brief period, at age 34, he became involved with a spinster who had fallen in love with him, but her family soon put an end to this relationship.

Thus, apart from some brief love associations with generally unattainable women, the only other heterosexual relationships known about are his relationships with prostitutes. He briefly lived with a girl called Christine in 1882, from whom he contracted gonorrhoea, and he was known to hang around brothels while at Arles. However, he suggested on more than one occasion that he only infrequently had sexual relationships with them and wrote to Theo of his impotence. It has been suggested that his association with prostitutes was related more to his and their mutual status as outcasts from society rather than necessarily as a means of sexual satisfaction.

SUMMARY

There is then evidence that van Gogh had episodes of an acute nature in which he became psychotic with bizarre delusions, hallucinations, and alternation of consciousness. It is suggested that these were ictal or postictal, possibly a complex partial seizure status. There is some substance to the suggestion that he had hypergraphia, hyperreligiosity, and was relatively asexual.

Gastaut also noted other evidence of a personality disorder. He was generally considered eccentric by those who knew him and apparently looked "perpetually undernourished." His moods were known to be volatile, ranging from the depths of depression to elation, and he was prone to violent outbursts of rage. These features and those listed above led Gastaut to the conclusion that van Gogh had psychomotor epilepsy with a medial temporal lobe focus.

SELECTED REFERENCES

Jaspers (1922), Riese (1925), Minkowska (1932), Gastaut (1956), Lubin (1975), Roskill (1986).

References

Abrahams, R., Taylor, M.A. Differential EEG patterns in affective disorder and schizophrenia. *Archives of General Psychiatry* 1979; 36:1355–1358.

Adamec, R.E. Kindling, anxiety and personality. In: T.G. Bolwig and M.R. Trimble eds. *The Clinical Relevance of Kindling*. J Wiley & Sons, Chichester, 1989; 117–135.

Adamec, R.E., Stark-Adamec, C. Limbic kindling and animal behaviour. *Biological Psychiatry* 1983; 18:269–293.

Adams, F. *The extant works of Aretaeus*. The Sydenham Society, London, 1856.

Adams, F. *The genuine works of Hippocrates*. Williams and Wilkins, Baltimore, 1939.

Albright, P.S., Burnham, W.I. Development of a new pharmacological seizure model: effects of anticonvulsants on cortical and amygdala-kindled seizures in the rat. *Epilepsia* 1980; 21:681–689.

Alheid, G.F., Heimer, L. New perspectives in basal forebrain organisation of special relevance for neuropsychiatric disorders. *Neuroscience* 1988; 27:1–39.

Alstrom, C.H. A study of epilepsy in its clinical, social, and genetic aspects. *Acta Psychiatra Scandanavica*, 1950; Suppl. 63.

American Psychiatric Association. Diagnostic and Statistical Manual of Mental Disorders (Third Edition). American Psychiatric Association, Washington D.C. 1980.

American Psychiatric Association. Diagnostic and Statistical Manual of Mental Disorders DSM-III-R. American Psychiatric Association, Washington D.C. 1987.

Aretaeus (see Adams, 1856).

Aschaffenberg, G. Über die Stimmungs-Schwankungen der Epileptiker. Marhold. Halle. 1906.

Asuni, T., Pillutla, V.S. Schizophrenia-like psychosis in Nigerian epileptics. *British Journal of Psychiatry* 1967; 113:1375–1379.

Babb, T. L., Brown, W. J., Pretorius, J., Davenport, C., Lieb, J.P., Crandall, P.H. Temporal lobe volumetric cell densities in temporal lobe epilepsy. *Epilepsia* 1984; 25:729–740.

Bailey, P., Gibbs, F.A. The surgical treatment of psychomotor epilepsy. *Journal of the American Medical Association* 1951; 145:365–500.

Barczak, P., Edmunds, E., Betts, T. Hypomania following complex partial seizures. *British Journal of Psychiatry* 1988; 152:137–139.

Barraclough, B. Suicide and epilepsy. In: E. H. Reynolds and M. R. Trimble, eds. *Epilepsy and Psychiatry*. Churchill Livingstone, Edinburgh, 1981; 72–76.

Bartlet, J.E.A. Chronic psychosis following epilepsy. *American Journal of Psychology* 1957; 114:338–343.

Bear, D.M., Fedio, P. Quantitative analysis of interictal behaviour in temporal lobe epilepsy. *Archives of Neurology* 1977; 34:454–467.

Bear, D.M., Levin, K., Blumer, D., Chetham, D., Ryder, J. Interictal behaviour in hospitalised temporal lobe epileptics: relationship to idiopathic psychiatric syndromes. *Journal of Neurology, Neurosurgery and Psychiatry* 1982; 45:481–488.

Beard, A.W. The schizophrenia-like psychoses of epilepsy. 2. Physical Aspects. *British Journal of Psychiatry* 1963; 109:113–129.

Bech, P., Pedersen, K.K., Simonsen, N., Lund, M. Personality traits in epilepsy. In: J. K. Penry, ed. *Epilepsy: The 8th International Symposium*. Raven Press, New York, 1977; 257–263.

Belenky, G., Tortella, F.C., Hitzeman, J., Holaday, J.W. The role of endorphin systems in the effects of ECS. In: B. Lerer, R. D. Weiner, and R. H. Belmaker, eds. *Basic Mechanisms*. J. Libbey, London, 1984; 89–97.

Ben-Ari, Y. Transmitters and modulators in the amygdaloid complex: a review. In: Y. Ben-Ari, ed. *The Amygdaloid Complex*. Elsevier, North Holland, 1981; 163–174.

Bergstrom, D.A., Kellar, K.J. Effects of ECS on monoaminergic receptor binding sites in rat brain. *Nature* 1979; 278:464–466.

Bernardi, S., Gallhofer, B., Trimble, M.R., Frackowiak, R.S.J., Wise, R.J.S., Jones, T. An interictal study of partial epilepsy using the oxygen-15 inhalation technique and PET with special reference to psychosis. In: *Current Problems in Epilepsy*, Vol. 1., J. Libby, London, 1984; 44–50.

Berrios, G. Insanity and epilepsy in the 19th century. In: M. Roth, and V. Cowie, eds. *Psychiatry, Genetics and Pathology*. Gaskal Press, London, 1979.

Besson, J.A.O., Corrigan, F.M., Cherryman, G.R., Smith, F.W. NMR in chronic schizophrenia. *British Journal of Psychiatry* 1987; 150:161–163.

Betts, T.A. A follow-up of a cohort of patients with epilepsy admitted to psychiatric care in an English city. In: P. Harris and C. Mawdsley, eds. *Epilepsy*. Churchill Livingstone, Edinburgh, 1974, 326–336.

Betts, T.A. Epilepsy and the mental hospital. In: E.H. Reynolds and M.R. Trimble, eds. *Epilepsy and Psychiatry*. Churchill Livingstone, Edinburgh, 1981; 175–184.

Betts, T., Kalra, P., Cooper, R., Jeavons, P. Epileptic fits as a probable side effect of amytriptyline. *Lancet* 1968; 1:390–392.

Bingley, T. Mental symptoms in temporal lobe epilepsy and temporal lobe gliomas. *Acta Psychiatrica Neurologica Scandinavica*, suppl 120, vol. 33, 1958.

Bleuler, E. *Dementia Praecox or the Group of Schizophrenics*, translated by J. Zenkin, 1950. International University Press: New York, 1911.

Bogerts, B., Hantsch, J., Herzer, M. A morphometric study of the dopamine-containing cell groups in the mesencephalon of normals, Parkinson patients and schizophrenics. *Archives of General Psychiatry* 1983; 18:951–970.

Bogerts, B., Meertz, E., Schonfeldt-Bausch, R. Basal ganglia and limbic system pathology in schizophrenia. *Archives of General Psychiatry* 1985; 42:784–791.

Bolwig, T.G., Trimble, M.R. *The Clinical Relevance of Kindling*. Wiley, Chichester, 1989.

Bonhoeffer, K. Zur Frage der exogenen Psychosen. *Zentrenblatt für Nervenkrankheiten* 1909; 32:499–505.

Bouchet, M., Cazauvieilh, M. De l'épilepsie considérée dans ses reapports avec l'aliénation mentale. *Archives Général de Medicine* 1825; 9:510–542; 10:5–50.

Boudin, G., Lauras, A., Tabary, J.C. La place de l'épilepsie dans la gènese des episodes psychotic: a propos de l'étude analytique de 27 observations personelles. *La Presse Medicale* 1963; 51:2431–2435.

Brandt, J., Seidman, L.J., Kohl, D. Personality characteristics of epileptic patients: a controlled study of generalized and temporal lobe cases. *Journal of Clinical and Experimental Neuropsychology* 1985; 7:25–38.

Bratz, H., Leubuscher, H. Die affekt-epilepsie. *Deutsche Medizinische Wochenschrift*. 1907; 33:592–593.

Broca, P. Anatomiè comparée des circonvolutions cérébrals: le grand lobe limbique et la scissure limbique dans la série des mammiferès. *Revue Anthropologie*, Serie 2, 1878; 1:385–498.

Brown, R., Colter, N., Corsellis, N., Crow, T.J., et al. Post-mortem evidence of structural brain changes in schizophrenia. *Archives of General Psychiatry* 1986; 43:36–42.

Bruens, J.H. Psychosis in Epilepsy. *Psychiatrica, Neurologica, Neurochirurgica* 1971; 74: 174–192.

Bruens, J.H. Psychoses in Epilepsy. In: P.J. Vinken and S.W. Bruyn, eds. *Handbook of clinical neurology*, vol. 15. North Holland Publishing Company, Amsterdam, 1974; 595–610.

Bruens, J.H. Different kinds of psychosis as related to different kinds of epilepsy. Presented at the study group of psychoses of epilepsy, 12th International Epilepsy Congress, Copenhagen, 1980.

Bruton, C.J. The neuropathology of temporal lobe epilepsy. In: *Maudsley Monograph No. 31*, Oxford University Press: Oxford, 1988.

Burckhardt, G. Ueber Rindenexcisionen als Beitrag zur operativen Therapie der Psychosen. Zeitschrift für Psychiatrie und psychisch-gerichtliche Medizin 1891; 47:463–548.

Byrne, A. Hypomania following increased epileptic activity. *British Journal of Psychiatry* 1988; 153:573–574.

Cairns, V.M. Epilepsy, Personality and Behaviour. In: P. Harris and C. Mawdsley, eds. *Epilepsy* Churchill Livingstone, Edinburgh, 1974; 256–263.

Cavanagh, J.B., Falconer, M.A., Mayer, A. Some pathogenic problems of temporal lobe epilepsy. In: Baldwin and P. Bailey, eds. *Temporal Lobe Epilepsy* Charles C. Thomas, Springfield, 1958; 140–148.

Christison, G.W., Casanova, M.F., Weinberger, D.R., Rawlings, R., Kleinman, J.E. A quantitative investigation of hippocampal pyramidal cell size, shape and variability of orientation in schizophrenia. *Archives of General Psychiatry* 1989; 46:1027–1032.

Clark, L.P. The psychobiological concept of essential epilepsy. *Journal of Nervous and Mental Disease* 1923; 57:433–444.

Clark, R.A., Lesko, J.M. Psychoses associated with epilepsy. *American Journal of Psychiatry* 1939; 96:595–607.

Clifford, D.B., Podolsky, A., Zorumski, C.F. Acute effects of Lithium on hippocampal kindled seizures. *Epilepsia* 1985; 26:689–692.

Clouston, T.S. *Clinical Lectures on Mental Diseases*, 4th edition. Churchill, London, 1896.

Conlon, P., Trimble, M.R., Rogers, D. A study of epileptic psychosis using M.R.I. *British Journal of Psychiatry* 1990; 156:231–235.

Conlon, P., Trimble, M.R., Rogers, D., Callicott, C. MRI in epilepsy: a controlled study. *Epilepsy Research* 1988; 2:37–43.

Coppen, A., Swade, S., Wood, K. Lithium restores abnormal platelet 5-HT transport in patients with affective disorders. *British Journal of Psychiatry* 1980; 136:235–238.

Costain, D.W., Gelder, M.G., Gwen, P.J., Grahame-Smith, D.G. ECT and the brain: evidence for increased dopamine-mediated responses. *Lancet* 1982; 2:400–404.

Crandall, P.H. Cortical resections. In: J. Engel, ed. *Surgical Treatment of the Epilepsies*. Raven Press, New York, 1987; 377–404.

Crow, T.J., Johnstone, E.C. Controlled trials of ECT. In: S. Malitz and H.A. Sackheim, eds. *ECT*, Annals of the New York Academy of Sciences 1986; 462:12–29.

Crow, T.J., Ball, J., Bloom, S.R., Brown, R., Bruton, C.J. et al. Schizophrenia as an anomaly of development of cerebral asymmetry. *Archives of General Psychiatry* 1989; 46:1145–1151.

Csernansky, J.G., Mellentin, J., Beauclair, L., Lombrozo, L. Mesolimbic dopaminergic supersensitivity following electrical kindling of the amygdala. *Biological Psychiatry* 1988; 23:285–294.

Cullen, W. *Nosology*. Creech, Edinburgh, 1800.

Curie, S., Heathfield, K.W.G., Henson, R.A., Scott, D. F. Clinical course and prognosis of TLE: a survey of 666 patients. *Brain* 1971; 94:173–190.

Curry, S.H., Davis, J.M., Janowsky, D.J., Marshall, J.H.L. Factors affecting chlorpromazine plasma levels in psychiatric patients. *Archives of General Psychiatry* 1970; 22:209–215.

Cutter, J.S. Benjamin W. Dudley and the surgical relief of traumatic epilepsy. *International Abstracts Surgery* 1930; 50:189–194.

Dam, A.M. Epilepsy and neurone loss in the hippocampus. *Epilepsia* 1980; 21:617–629.

Dana-Haeri, J., Trimble, M.R. Prolactin and gonadotrophin changes following partial seizures in epileptic patients with and without psychopathology. *Biological Psychiatry* 1984; 19:329–336.

Davison, K., Bagley, C.R. Schizophrenia-like psychoses associated with organic disorders of the CNS: a review of the literature. In: R.N. Herrington, ed. *Current Problems in Neuropsychiatry* Headley Brothers, Kent, 1969; 133–184.

Delgado, J.M.R. Aggressive behaviour evoked by radio stimulation in monkey colonies. *American Zoologist* 1966; 6:660–681.

DeLisi, L.E., Buchsbaum, M.S., Holocomb, H.H., Langston, K.C., King, A.C. et al. Increased temporal lobe glucose use in chronic schizophrenic patients. *Biological Psychiatry* 1989; 25:835–851.

Demers, J., Lukesh, R., Prichard, J. Convulsion during lithium therapy. *Lancet* 1970; 2:315–316.

Dewhurst, K., Beard, A.W. Sudden religious conversions in temporal lobe epilepsy. *British Journal of Psychiatry* 1970; 117:497–507.

Dikmen, S., Hermann, B.P., Wilensky, A.J., Rainwater, G. Validity of the MMPI to psychopathology in patients with epilepsy. *Journal of Nervous and Mental Disease* 1983; 171:114–122.

Dodrill, C.D. Neuropsychology. In: J. Laidlaw, A. Richens, and J. Oxley, eds. *A textbook of Epilepsy* Churchill Livingstone, Edinburgh 1988; 406–420.

Dongier, S. Statistical study of clinical and EEG manifestations of 536 psychotic episodes occurring in 516 epileptics between clinical seizures. *Epilepsia* 1959, 1960; 1:117–142.

Dorr-Zegers, O., Rauh, J. Different kinds of psychoses as related to different kinds of epilepsy. Presented at study group of psychoses of epilepsy, 12th International Epilepsy Congress, Copenhagen, 1980.

Dyve, S., Sherwin, A., Gjedde, A. Dopamine synthesis in unilateral temporal lobe epilepsy determined with 6-18F Fluorodopa. [Abstract] presented at the British Association for Psychopharmacology Summer meeting, No. 63. Cambridge, England, 1989.

Earle, K.M., Baldwin, M., Penfield, W. Incisural sclerosis and temporal lobe seizures produced by hippocampal herniation at birth. *Archives of Neurology and Psychiatry* 1953; 69:27–42.

Echeverria, M.G. On epileptic insanity. *American Journal of Insanity* 1873; 301–351.

Edeh, J., Toone, B. Relationship between interictal psychopathology and the type of epilepsy. *British Journal of Psychiatry* 1987; 151:95–101.

Ellis, J.M., Lee, S.I. Acute prolonged confusion in later life as an ictal state. *Epilepsia* 1978; 19:199–128.

Engel, J. *The Surgical Treatment of the Epilepsies.* Raven Press, New York, 1987.

Engel, J., Ludwig, B., Fetell, M. Prolonged partial complex status epilepticus: EEG and behavioural observations. *Neurology* 1978; 28:862–869.

Ervin, F., Epstein, A.W., King, H.E. Behaviour of epileptic and non-epileptic patients with temporal spikes. *Archives of Neurology and Psychiatry* 1955; 74:488–497.

Esquirol, J. Mental maladies: a treatise on insanity. Translated by E.K. Hunt. Lea and Blanchard, Philadelphia, 1845.

Faber, R., Trimble, M.R. *ECT and Parkinson's Disease,* in press, 1991.

Falconer, M. Discussion. In: M. Baldwin and P. Bailey, eds. *Temporal Lobe Epilepsy* Charles C. Thomas, Springfield, 1958; 537–558.

Falconer, M.A. Reversibility by temporal lobe resection of the behaviour abnormalities of temporal lobe epilepsy. *New England Journal of Medicine* 1963; 289:451–455.

Falconer, M.A., Taylor, D.C. Surgical treatment of drug resistant epilepsy due to mesial temporal sclerosis. *Archives of Neurology* 1968; 19:353–361.

Falkai, P., Bogerts, B., Rozumek, M. Limbic pathology in schizophrenia. The entorhinal region—a morphometric study. *Biological Psychiatry* 1988; 24:515–521.

Falret, J. D' l'état mental des épileptiques. *Archives Générales de Médecine* 1860, 1861; 16:661–699; 17:461–491; 18:423–443.

Feighner, J.P., Robins, E., Guze, S.B., Woodruff, R.A., Winokur, G., Munoz, R. Diagnostic criteria for use in psychiatric research. *Archives of General Psychiatry* 1972; 26:57–63.

Feinstein, A., Ron, M.A. Psychosis associated with demonstrable disease of the CNS. *Psychological Medicine,* in press, 1990.

Fenton, G.W. Epilepsy and Psychosis. *Journal of the Irish Medical Association* 1978; 71:315–324.

Fenwick, P.B.C. Postscript: What should be included in a standard psychiatric assessment. In: J. Engel, ed. *Surgical Treatment of the Epilepsies* Raven Press, New York, 1987; 505–510.

Ferguson, S.M., Rayport, M. Living with Epilepsy. *Journal of Nervous and Mental Disease* 1965; 140:26–37.

Ferriar, J. *Medical Histories and Relections.* Cadell and Davies, London, 1795.

Ferrier, I.N., Crow, T.J., Roberts, G.W. et al. Alterations in neuropeptides in the limbic lobe in schizophrenia. In: M.R. Trimble and E. Zarifian, eds. *Psychopharmacology of the Limbic System.* Oxford University Press, Oxford, 1984; 244–254.

Fischer, M., Korskjeer, G., Pederson, E. Psychotic episodes with Zaronden treatment. *Epilepsia* 1965; 6:325–334.

Flor-Henry, P. Psychosis and Temporal Lobe Epilepsy. *Epilepsia* 1969; 10:363–395.

Forrest, F.M., Forrest, I.S., Serra, M.T. Modification of chlorpromazine metabolism by some other drugs frequently administered to psychiatric patients. *Biological Psychiatry* 1970; 2:53–58.

Freud, S. Dostoevsky and Parricide. In: J. Strachey, ed. *Sigmund Freud Collected papers* Hogarth, London, 1953; 5:222–242.

Fulton, J.F. Discussion. *Epilepsia* 1953; 2:77.

Fuster, J.M. *The Prefrontal Cortex.* Raven Press, New York, 1980.

Gallhofer, B., Trimble, M.R., Frackowiak, R., Gibbs, J., Jones, T. A study of cerebral blood flow and metabolism in epileptic psychosis using PET and oxygen-15. *Journal of Neurology, Neurosurgery and Psychiatry,* 1985: 48;201–206.

Garryfallos, G., Manos, N., Adamobulou, A. Psychopathology and personality characteristics of epileptic patients. *Acta Psychiatrica Scandinavica* 1988; 78:87–95.

Gastaut, H. Etude électroclinique des épisodes psychotiques survenant en dehors des crises cliniques chez les épileptiques. *Revue Neurologie* 1956; 94:587–594.

Gastaut, H. La maladie de Vincent Van Gogh. *Annales Médico Psychologiques* 1956; 114:196–238.

Gastaut, H. Fyodor Mikhailovitch Dostoevsky's involuntary contribution to the symptomatology and prognosis of epilepsy. *Epilepsia* 1978; 19:186–201.

Gastaut, H., Roger, J., Lefevre, N. Différenciation psychologique des épileptiques en fonction des formes électrocliniques de leur maladie. *Revue Psychologique,* App. 1953; 3:237–249.

Gaupp. Zur Frage der Kombinierten psychosen. *Zentralblatt für Nervenheilkunde und Psychiatrie* 1903; 26; 766–775.

Gibberd, F.B., Dunne, J.F., Handley, A.J., Hazelman, B.L. Supervision of epileptic patients taking phenytoin. *British Medical Journal* 1970; 1:147–149.

Gibbs, F.A. Ictal and Non-ictal psychiatric disorders in temporal lobe epilepsy. *Journal of Nervous and Mental Disease* 1951; 113:522–528.

Gibbs, F.A., Gibbs, E.L. *Atlas of Electroencephalography*. Addison-Wesley, Cambridge, Mass., 1952.

Gibbs, F.A., Gibbs, E.L., Lennox, W.G. The likeness of the cortical dysrhythmias of schizophrenia and psychomotor epilepsy. *American Journal of Psychiatry* 1936; 95:255–269.

Gibbs, F.A., Gibbs, E.L., Lennox, W.G. Epilepsy: a paroxysmal cerebral dysrhythmia. *Brain* 1937; 60:377–388.

Gibbs, F.A., Gibbs, E.L., Lennox, W.G. Cerebral dysrhythmias of epilepsy *Archives of Neurology and Psychiatry* 1938; 39:298–314.

Gibbs, F.A., Stamps, F.W. *Epilepsy Handbook*. Thomas, Springfield, 1953.

Gillig, P., Sackellares, J.C., Greenberg, H.P. Right hemisphere partial complex seizures. *Epilepsia* 1988; 29:26–29.

Girgis, M. *Neural Substrates of Limbic Epilepsy*. Warren H. Green, Missouri, 1981.

Glaser, G.H. The problem of psychosis in psychomotor temporal lobe epileptics. *Epilepsia* 1964; 5:271–278.

Glaser, G.H. Limbic epilepsy in childhood. *Journal of Nervous and Mental Disease* 1967; 144:391–397.

Glaus, A. Ueeber Kombinationen von Schizophrenie und Epilepsie. *Zeitschrift für die gesamte Neurologie und Psychiatrie* 1931; 135:450–500.

Glitheroe, E., Slater, E. Follow up record and outcome. *British Journal of Psychiatry* 1963; 109:134–142.

Gloor, P. Neurobiological substrates of ictal behavioural changes. In: D. Smith, D. Treiman and M.R. Trimble, eds. *Neurobehavioral Problems in Epilepsy*. Raven Press, New York, 1991; 1–34.

Gloor, P., Oliver, A., Quesney, L.F., Andermann, F., Horowitz, S. The role of the limbic system in experiential phenomena of temporal lobe epilepsy. *Annals of Neurology* 1982; 12:129–144.

Goldberg, L.R. Man versus mean. *Journal of Abnormal Psychology* 1972; 79:121–131.

Goodwin, D.W., Guze, S.B. *Psychiatric Diagnoses*, third edition. Oxford University Press, Oxford, 1984.

Gowers, W.R. *Epilepsy and Other Chronic Convulsive Diseases*. Churchill, London, 1901.

Grahame-Smith, D.G., Green, A.R., Costain, D.W. Mechanism of action of ECT. *Lancet* 1978; 1:245–256.

Gray, J.G. *The Neuropsychology of Anxiety* Oxford University Press, Oxford, 1982.

Graybiel, A.M. Neurochemically specified subsystems in the basal ganglia. In: D. Evered and M. O'Conner, eds. *Functions of the Basal Ganglia* Pitman, London, 1984; 114–143.

Green, J.R., Duwberg, R.E.H., McGrath, W.B. Focal epilepsy of psychomotor type. *Journal of Neurosurgery* 1951; 8:157–172.

Griesinger, W. *Mental Pathology and Therapeutics*. New Sydenham Society, London, 1857.

Grignotta, F., Todesco, C.V., Lugaresi, E. Temporal lobe epilepsy with ecstatic seizures. *Epilepsia* 1980; 21:705–710.

Gudmundsson, G. Epilepsy in Iceland. *Acta Neurologica Scandinavica*, suppl. 25, 1966.

Guerrant, J., Anderson, W.W., Fischer, A., Weinstein, M.R., Jaros, R.M., Deskins, A. *Personality in Epilepsy*. Thomas, Springfield, 1962.

Gupta, A.K., Jeavous, P.M., Hughes, R.C., Covanis, A. Aura in temporal lobe epilepsy: clinical and EEG correlation. *Journal of Neurology, Neurosurgery and Psychiatry* 1983; 46:1079–1083.

Gur, R.E., Gur, R.C., Skolnic, B., Caroff, S., Obrist, W.D., Reswick, S., Reivich, M. Brain function in psychiatric disorders III. rCBF in unmedicated schizophrenics. *Archives of General Psychiatry* 1985; 42:329–334.

Halgren, E., Warter, R.D., Cherlois, D.G., Crandall, P.H. Mental phenomena evoked by electrical stimulation of the human hippocampal formation and amygdala. *Brain* 1978; 101:83–118.

Hara, T., Hoshi, A., Takase, M., Sato, S. Factors related to psychiatric episodes in epileptics. *Folia Psychiatrica et Neurologica Japonica* 1980; 34:329–330.

Harle, J. An historial essay on the state of physick in the old and new testament and the apocryphal interval. London, 1729.

Heath, R.G. Common clinical characteristics of epilepsy and schizophrenia. *American Journal of Psychiatry* 1962; 11:1013–1026.

Heath, R.G. Pleasure and brain activity in man. *Journal of Nervous and Mental Disease* 1972; 154:3–18.

Heath, R.G., Brain function and behaviour. *Journal of Nervous and Mental Disease* 1975; 60:159–175.

Heath, R.G. Psychosis and epilepsy: similarities and differences in the anatomic-physiologic substrait. In: W. P. Koella and M.R. Trimble, eds. *Temporal lobe epilepsy, mania and schizophrenia and the limbic system* Karger, Basel, 1982; 106–116.

Heimer, L., Larsson, E. Impairment of mating behaviour in male rats following lesions in the pre-optic and anterior hypothalamic continuum. *Brain Research* 1966; 3:248–263.

Heimer, L., Switzer, R.D., Van Hoesen, G.W. Ventral striatum and ventral pallidum. *Trends in Neurosciences* 1982; 5:83–87.

Helgason, R. Epidemiology of mental disorders in Iceland. *Acta Psychiatrica Scandinavica*, supp. 142, 1964.

Hendley, E.D., Welch, B.L. ECS: sustained decrease in norepinephrine uptake affinity in a reserpine model of depression. *Life Science* 1975; 16:45–54.

Herbert, J. Behaviour and the limbic system with particular reference to sexual and aggressive interactions. In: M. R. Trimble and E. Zarifian, eds. *Psychopharmacology of the Limbic System* Oxford University Press, Oxford, 1984; 51–67.

Hermann, B.P., Dikmen, S., Schwartz, M.S., Karnes, W.E. Interictal psychopathology in patients with ictal fear: a quantitative investigation. *Neurology* 1982; 32:7–11.

Hermann, B.P., Dikmen, S., Wilensky, A. Increased psychopathology associated with multiple seizure types: fact or artefact. *Epilepsia* 1982; 23:587–598.

Hermann, B.P., Riel, P. Interictal personality and behaviour traits in temporal lobe and generalised epilepsy. *Cortex* 1981; 17:125–128.

Hermann, B.P., Schwartz, M.S., Karnes, W.E., Valdat, P. Psychopathology in epilepsy: relationship of seizure type to age of onset. *Epilepsia* 1980; 21:15–23.

Hermann, B.P., Wyler, A.R. Effects of anterior lobectomy on language function: a controlled study. *Annals of Neurology* 1988; 23:585–588.

Herpin, T.H. *Du prognostic et du traitement curatif de L'épilepsie*. Baillière, Paris, 1852.

Hill, D. Psychiatry. In: D. Hill and G. Parr, eds. *Electroencephalography*, MacDonald, London, 1950; 319–363.

Hill, D. Psychiatric disorders of epilepsy. *The Medical Press* 1953; 229:473–475.

Hill, D. Troubles psychologiques intercritiques chez les épileptics. *Revue Neurologique* 1956; 95:608.

Hill, D. Historical review, epilepsy and psychiatry. In: E.H. Reynolds, M.R. Trimble, eds. *Epilepsy and Psychiatry*. Churchill Livingstone, Edinburgh, 1981; 1–11.

Hill, D., Pond, D.W., Mitchell, W., Falconer, M.A. Personality changes following temporal lobectomy for epilepsy. *Journal of Mental Science* 1957; 103:18–27.

Hippocrates—see Adams, F., 1939.

Hoch, P.J. Clinical and biological interrelations between schizophrenia and epilepsy. *American Journal of Psychiatry* 1943; 100:507–512.

Hoffmann, H. See Aschaffenberg, 1906.

Horsley, V. Brain Surgery. *British Medical Journal* 1886; Oct:670–675.

Howden, J.C. The religious sentiments of epileptics. *Journal of Mental Science* 1872, 1873; 18:491–497.

Hunter, R.A. Status epilepticus: history, incidence and problems. *Epilepsia* 1959, 1960; 1:162–188.

Hurwitz, T.A., Wada, J.A., Kosaka, B.D., Strauss E. Cerebral organisation of affect suggested by temporal lobe seizures. *Neurology* 1985; 35:1335–1337.

International League Against Epilepsy: Proposal for revised clinical and electroencephalographic classification of epileptic seizures. *Epilepsia* 1981; 22:489–501.

International League Against Epilepsy. Proposal for classification of the epilepsies and epileptic syndromes. *Epilepsia* 1985; 26:268–278.

Isaacson, R.L. *The Limbic System*, second edition. Plenum Press, New York, 1982.

Itil, T.M. Convulsive and anticonvulsive properties of neuro-psychopharmaca. *Modern Problems of Pharmacopsychiatry* 1970; 4:270–300.

Iversen, S. Behavioural Effects of Manipulation of Basalganglia Neurotransmitter. In: D. Evered, M. O'Connor, eds. *Functions of the Basalganglia*. Pittman, London, 1984; 183–195.

Jackson, J.H. On temporary mental disorders after epileptic paroxysms. *West Riding Lunatic Asylum Medical Reports* 1875; 5:105–129.

Jackson, J.H. On temporary mental disorders after epileptic paroxysms. *West Riding Lunatic Asylum Medical Reports* 1875; 5:105–129.

Jackson, J.H. Lecturers on the diagnosis of epilepsy. *Medical Times and Gazette* 1879; 1:141–143.

Jackson, J.H. On right or left-sided spasm at the onset of epileptic paroxysms, and on crude sensation warnings and elaborate mental states. *Brain* 1880, 1881; 3:192–206.

Jackson, J.H. On temporary paralysis after epileptiform and epileptic seizures. *Brain* 1880, 1881; 3:433–451.

Jackson. J.H. The factors of Insanities. *Medical Press and Circular* 1894; 2:615–619.

Jakob, H., Beckmann, H. Gross and histological criteria for developmental disorders in brains of schizophrenics. *Journal of the Royal Society of Medicine* 1989; 82:466–469.

Janicak, P.G., Easton, M.S., Comaty, J.E., Dowd, S., David, J.M. Efficacy of ECT in psychotic and non-psychotic depression. *Convulsive Therapy* 1989; 5:314–320.

Jann, M.W., Ereshefsky, L., Saklad, S.K. et al. Effects of carbamazepine on plasma haloperidol levels. *Journal of Clinical Psychopharmacology* 1985; 2:106–143.

Jasper, H.H., Fitzpatrick, G.P., Solomon, P. Analogies and opposites in schizophrenia and epilepsy. *American Journal of Psychiatry* 1939; 65:835–850.

Jasper, H.H., Pertuiset, B., Flanigin, H. EEG and cortical electrograms in patients with temporal lobe seizures. *Archives of Neurology and Psychiatry* 1951; 65:272–290.

Jaspers, K. *General Psychopathology* (1922), translated by J. Hoenig and M.W. Hamilton. Manchester University Press, Manchester, 1963.

Jaspers, K. Van Gogh and schizophrenia. In: B. Welsh-Ovcharov, ed. *Van Gogh in perspective*. Prentice Hall, New Jersey 1974; 99–101.

Jensen, I. Temporal lobe surgery around the world. *Acta Neurologica Scandinavica* 1975; 52:354–373.

Jensen, I., Larsen, J.K. Mental aspects of temporal lobe epilepsy. *Journal of Neurology, Neurosurgery and Psychiatry* 1979; 42:256–265.

Jensen, I., Larsen, J.K. Psychoses in drug resistant temporal lobe epilepsy. *Journal of Neurology, Neurosurgery and Psychiatry* 1979; 42:948–954.

Jensen, I., Vaernet, K. Temporal lobe epilepsy: Follow-up investigation of temporal lobe resected patients. *Acta Neurologica Scandinavica* 1977; 37:173–200.

Jeste, D.V., Lohr, J.B. Hippocampal pathologic findings in schizophrenia. *Archives of General Psychiatry* 1989; 46:1019–1024.

Johannsson, O., Hokfelt, T. Nucleus accumbens: transmitter neurochemistry with special reference to peptide containing neurones. In: R. B. Chronister and J. F. DeFrance, eds. *The neurobiology of the nucleus accumbens* Haer Institute, Brunswick, 1981; 147–172.

Johnstone, E.C., Deakin, J.F.W., Lawler, P., Frith, C.D., Stevens, M., McPherson, K., Crow, T.J. The Northwick Park ECT trial. *Lancet* 1980; 2:1317–1320.

Johnstone, E.C., Owens, D.G.C., Crow, T.J., Frith, C.D., Alexandropolis, K., Bydder, G., Colter, W. Temporal lobe structure as determined by nuclear magnetic resonance in schizophrenia and bipolar affective disorder. *Journal of Neurology, Neurosurgery and Psychiatry* 1989; 52:736–741.

Jones, E.G., Powell, T.P.S. An anatomical study of converging sensory pathways within the cerebral cortex of the monkey. *Brain* 1970; 93:793–820.

Jorgensen, R.S., Wulff, M.H. The effect of orally administered chlorpromazine on the EEG in man. *Electroencephalography and Clinical Neurophysiology* 1958; 10:325–329.

Jus, A. Troubles mentaux a symptomatalogie schizophrénique chez les épileptiques. *Evolution and Psychiatry* 1966; 31:313–319.

Juul-Jensen, P. Epilepsy. *Acta Neurologica Scandinavica*, Supp. 5, 1964; 40:1–148.

Kamm, I., Mandel, A. Thioridazine in the treatment of behaviour disorders in epileptics. *Diseases of the Nervous System* 1967; 28:46–48.

Kanaka, T.S., Balasubramaniam, V., Ramamurthi, B. Mental changes in epilepsy. *Neurology* (India) 1966; 15:113–118.

Kanemoto, K., Janz, D. The temporal sequence of aura-sensations in patients with complex focal seizures with particular attention to ictal aphasia. *Journal of Neurology, Neurosurgery and Psychiatry* 1989; 52:52–56.

Karagulla, S., Robertson, E.E. Psychical phenomena in temporal lobe epilepsy. *British Medical Journal* 1955; 1:748–752.

Kendrick, J.F., Gibbs, F.A. Origin, spread and neurological treatment of the psychomotor type of seizure discharge. *Journal of Neurosurgery* 1957; 14:270–284.

Kenwood, C., Betts, T. 20 year follow-up of epileptic psychosis. *British, Danish, Dutch, Epilepsy Congress Abstracts*, p. 53. Heemstede, Netherlands, 1988.

Kiloh, L., Davison, R., Osselton, J. An EEG study of the analeptic effects of imipramine. *Electroencephalography and Clinical Neurophysiology* 1961; 13:216–223.

Kling, A., Orbach, J., Schwartz, N.B., Towne, J.C. Injury to the limbic system and associated structures in cats. *Archives of General Psychiatry* 1960; 3:391–420.

Kløve, H., Doehring, H. MMPI in epileptic groups with differential aetiology. *Journal of Clinical Psychology* 1962; 18:149–153.

Klüver, H., Bucy, P.C. Preliminary analysis of functions of the temporal lobe in monkeys. *Archives of Neurology and Psychiatry* 1939; 42:979–1000.

Koehler, K. First rank symptoms of schizophrenia: questions concerning clinical boundaries. *British Journal of Psychiatry* 1979; 134:236–248.

Koella, W. The functions of the limbic system—evidence from animal experimentation. In: W. Koella and M.R. Trimble, eds. *Temporal Lobe Epilepsy, Mania, and Schizophrenia and the Limbic System* Karger, Basel, 1982; 12–39.

Kogeorgos, J., Fonagy, P., Scott, D.F. Psychiatric symptom profiles of chronic epileptics attending a neurological clinic: a controlled investigation. *British Journal of Psychiatry* 1982; 140:236–243.

Kovelman, J.A., Scheibel, A.B. A neurohistological correlate of schizophrenia. *Biological Psychiatry* 1984; 19:1601–1622.

Kraepelin, E. Lectures on Clinical Psychiatry. William Wood, New York, 1904.

Krapf, E. Epilepsie und Schizophrenie. *Archive fur Psychiatrie und Nervenkrank* 1928; 83:547–586.

Kristensen, O., Sindrup, E.H. Psychomotor epilepsy and psychosis. 1. Physical Aspects. *Acta Neurologica Scandinavica* 1978; 57:361–369.

Kristensen, O., Sindrup, E.H. Psychomotor epilepsy and psychosis. II. EEG findings. *Acta Neurologica Scandinavica* 1978; 57:370–379.

Kristensen, O., Sindrup, E.H. Psychomotor epilepsy and psychosis. III. Social and psychological correlates. *Acta Neurologica Scandinavica* 1979; 59:1–9.

Kutt, H., Haynes, J., McDowell, F. Some causes of ineffectiveness of DPH. *Archives of Neurology* 1966; 14:489–492.

Lai, C.W., Lai, Y.H.C. History of epilepsy in Chinese Traditional Medicine, in press, 1990.

Lamprecht, F. Biochemische Aspekte in der Psychsenforschung. In: H. Penin, ed. *Psychische Störungen bei Epilepsie*. Schattaner Verlag, Stuttgart, 1973; 85–105.

Landolt, H. Some clinical EEG correlations in epileptic psychoses (twilight states). *EEG and Clinical Neurophysiology* 1953; 5:121.

Landolt, H. Serial EEG investigations during psychotic episodes in epileptic patients and during schizophrenic attacks. In: A.M. Lorentz De Haas, ed. *Lectures on Epilepsy* Elsevier, Amsterdam, 1958; 91–133.

Landolt, H. Die Dämmer-und Verstimmungszustände bei Epilepsie und Ihre EEG. *Deutsche Zeitschrift für Nervenheilkunde* 1963; 185:411–430.

Landsborough, D. St Paul and temporal lobe epilepsy. *Journal of Neurology, Neurosurgery and Psychiatry* 1987; 50:659–665.

Larsby, H., Lindgren, E. Encephalographic examination of 125 institutionalised epileptics. *Acta Psychiatricia et Neurologica* 1940; 15:337–352.

Lennox, W.G., Cobb, S. Aura in epilepsy: a statistical review of 1359 cases. *Archives of Neurology and Psychiatry* 1933; 30:374–387.

Lennox, W.G., Lennox, M.A. See Guerrant et al., 1962.

Lennox, W.G., Lennox, M.A. *Epilepsy and Related Disorders*. Churchill, London, 1960.

Levin, S. Epileptic clouded states. *Journal of Nervous and Mental Disease* 1952; 116:215–225.

Lewis, A. Paranoia and paranoid: a historical perspective. *Psychological Medicine* 1952; 1:2–12.

Lewis, A. Endogenous and exogenous—a useful dichotomy. *Psychological Medicine* 1971; 1:191–196.

Lewis, A.J. Melancholia: a historical review. *Journal of Mental Science* 1934; 80:1–42.

Leysen, J., Niemegeers, C.J.E. Neuroleptics. In: A. Lagtha, ed. *Handbook of Neurochemistry*, Vol. 9. Plenum, New York, 1985; 331–361.

Liddell, D.W. (1953): Observations on epileptic automatism in a mental hospital population. *Journal of Mental Science*, 99:732–748.

Linnoila, M., Viukari, M., Vaisanen, K., Auvinen, J. (1980): Effects of anticonvulsants on plasma haloperidol and thioridazine levels. *American Journal of Psychiatry*, 137:819–821.

Lloyd, K.G., Bossi, L., Morselli, P.L., Rougier, M., Loiseau, P., Munari, C. Biochemical evidence for dysfunction of GABA neurones in human epilepsy. In: G. Bartholini, L. Bossi, K.G. Lloyd, and P.L. Morselli, eds. *Epilepsy and GABA receptor agonists*. Raven Press, New York, 1985; 43–51.

Lloyd, K.G., Thuret, F., Pilc, A. Upregulation of GABA binding sites in rat frontal cortex: a common action of repeated administration of different classes of anti-depressants and electroshock. *Journal of Pharmacology and Experimental Therapeutics* 1985; 235:191–199.

Logothetis, J. Spontaneous epileptic seizures and EEG changes in the course of phenothiazine therapy. *Neurology* 1967; 17:869–877.

Logsdail, S.J., Toone, B.K. Post-ictal Psychoses. *British Journal of Psychiatry* 1988; 152:246–252.

Long, J.B., Tortella, F.C. CSF from convulsed rats causes a naloxone reversible increase of seizure threshold of recipient animals. [Abstracts,] Society of Neuroscience, 145th Annual Meeting, No. 273, 1984; p. 929.

Lubin, A.J. *Stranger on earth: the life of Vincent Van Gogh*. Paladin, 1975.

Lugaresi, E., Pazzaglia, P., Tassinari, C.A. Differentiation of 'absence status' and temporal lobe status. *Epilepsia* 1971; 12:77–87.

MacCallum, W.A.G. Interaction of lithium and phenytoin. *British Medical Journal* 1980; 1:610–611.

Mace, C., Trimble, M. R. Post-operative psychoses following epilepsy surgery. *Journal of Neurology, Neurosurgery and Psychiatry (in press)*, 1991.

MacLean, P. D. Contrasting functions of limbic and neocortical systems of the brain and their relevance to psychophysiological aspects of medicine. *American Journal of Medicine* 1958; 25:611–626.

MacLean, P.D. The triune brain, emotion and scientific bias. In: F.O. Schmidt and F.G. Worden, eds. *The Neurosciences, Second Study Program*, Rockefeller University Press, New York, 1970; 336–349.

MacLean, P.D. The triune brain in evolution. Plenum, New York, 1990.

MacLean, P.D., Ploog, D.W. Cerebral representation of penile erection. *Journal of Neurophysiology* 1962; 25:29–55.

Maletzky, B. M. Seizure duration and clinical effect in psychiatry. *Comprehensive Psychiatry* 1978; 19:541–550.

Mann, S., Cree, W. New longer stay psychiatric patients. *Psychological Medicine* 1976; 6:603–616.

Marchand, L., De Ajuriaguerra, J. *Epilepsies*. Descleé de Brouwer and Cie, Paris, 1948.

Margerison, J.H., Corsellis, J. Epilepsy and the temporal lobes. *Brain* 1966; 89:499–530.

Master, D.R., Toone, B.K., Scott, D.F. Interictal behaviour in TLE. In: R. Porter, ed. *Advances in Epileptiology: 15th Epilepsy International Symposium* Raven Press, New York, 1984; 557–565.

Matthews, C.H.G., Kløve, H. MMPI performances in major motor, psychomotor and mixed seizure classifications of known and unknown aetiology. *Epilepsia* 1968; 9:43–53.

Maudsley, H. *Responsibility in Mental Disease*. Henry King, London, 1874.

Maudsley, H. *Body and Mind*. Appleton, New York, 1879.

Mayeux, J., Brandt, J., Rosen, J., Benson, F. Interictal memory and language in TLE. *Neurology* 1980; 30:120–125.

McCarley, R.W., Faux, S.F., Shenton, M., Le May, M., Cane, M., Ballinger, R., Duffy, F.H. CT abnormalities in schizophrenia. *Archives of General Psychiatry* 1989; 46:698–708.

McGuffin, P., Farmer, A.E., Gottesman, I., Murray, R.M., Reveley, A.M. Twin concordance for operationally defined schizophrenia. *Archives of General Psychiatry* 1984; 41:541–554.

McMillan, T.M., Powell, G.E., Janota, I., Polkey, C. Relationships between neuropathology and cognitive functioning in temporal lobectomy patients. *Journal of Neurology, Neurosurgery and Psychiatry* 1987; 50:167–176.

Mead, R. De Imperio Solis Ac Lunae in Corpora Humani, et Morbis inde Oriundis. London, 1746.

Meduna, L.V. Versuche über die biologische Beeinflussung des Ablaufs der Schizophrenie. *Zeitschrift für die gesamte Neurologie und Psychiatrie* 1935; 152:235–262.

Meduna, L.V. *Die Konvulsion therapie der schizophrenie*. Marhold, Halle, (1937).

Meduna, L.V. Il trattamento della schizofrenia negli Ospedali di state. *Rassegna di Studi Psichiatrici* 1938; 27, 883–896.

Meduna, L.V. Autobiography of L.J. Meduna. *Convulsive Therapy* 1985; 1:43–57.

Meier, M., French, L.A. Some personality correlates of unilateral and bilateral EEG abnormalities in psychomotor epileptics. *Journal of Clinical Psychology*, 1965; 21:3–9.

Meldrum, B.S. Pathophysiology of chronic epilepsy. In: M.R. Trimble, ed. *The Prognosis and Management of Resistant Epilepsy* Wiley, Chichester, 1989; 1–12.

Meldrum, B., Anlezark, G., Trimble, M.R. Drugs modifying dopaminergic activity and behaviour, the EEG and epilepsy in Papio papio. *European Journal of Pharmacology* 1975; 32:203–215.

Meldrum, B.S., Griffiths, T., Evans, M.C. Epileptic brain damage. In: F. Clifford-Rose, ed. *Research Progress in Epilepsy* Pitman, London, 1983; 78–86.

Mellanby, J. Kindling, Behaviour and Memory. In: *The Clinical Relevance of Kindling*, T.G. Bolwig and M.R. Trimble. eds. Wiley, Chichester, 1989; 103–112.

Mellor, C.S. First rank symptoms of schizophrenia. *British Journal of Psychiatry* 1970; 117:15–23.

Mendez, M.F., Cummings, J.L., Benson, D.F. Psychotropic drugs and epilepsy. *Stress Medicine* 1986; 2:325–332.

Mignone, R.J., Donnelly, E.F., Sadowsky, D. Psychological and Neurological Comparisons of psychomotor and non-psychomotor epileptic patients. *Epilepsia* 1970; 2:345–349.

Milner, B. Amnesia following operation on the temporal lobes. In: C.W.M. Whitty and O. L. Zangwill, eds. *Amnesia* Butterworths, London, 1966; 109–133.

Minkowska, F. Van Gogh as an epileptic. In: K. Jaspers, ed. *Strindberg und Van Gogh*. Bircher, Leipzig, 1932.

Mogenson, G.L. Jones, P.L., Yim, C.Y. From motivation to action: functional interface between the limbic system and the motor system. *Progress in Neurobiology* 1980; 14:69–97.

Morel, B.A. Traitè des maladies mentales. Paris, 1860.

Mulder, D.W., Daly, D. Psychiatric symptoms associated with lesions of the temporal lobes. *Journal of the American Medical Association* 1952; 150:173–176.

Mungas, D. Interictal behaviour abnormality in TLE. *Archives of General Psychiatry* 1982; 39:108–111.

Musacchio, J.M., Julou, K., Kety, S.S., Glowinski, J. Increase in rat brain tyrosine hydrolase activity produced by ECS. *Proceedings of the National Academy of Sciences* 1969; 63:1117–1119.

Nakajima, T., Post, R.M., Pert, A., Ketter, T.A., Weiss, S.R. Perspective on the mechanism of action of ECT. *Convulsive Therapy* 1989; 5:274–295.

Nauta, W.T.H. Some efferent connections of the pre-frontal cortex in the monkey. In: J.M. Warren and K. Akert, eds. *The frontal granular cortex and behavior* McGraw-Hill, New York, 1964;1397–1407.

Nauta, W.T.H., Domesick, V.B. Neural associations of the limbic system. In: A. Beckman, ed. *The neural Basis of Behaviour* Spectrum, New York, 1982; 175–206.

Nielsen, H., Kristensen, O. Personality correlates of sphenoidal EEG foci in temporal lobe epilepsy. *Acta Neurologica Scandinavica* 1981; 64:289–300.

Niemeyer, P. The transventricular amygdala-hippocampectomy in temporal lobe epilepsy. In: M. Baldwin and P. Bailey, eds. *Temporal Lobe Epilepsy* Thomas, Springfield, 1958; 461–482.

Nieto, D., Escobar, A. Major psychoses. In: J. Minkler, ed. *Pathology of the Nervous System*, vol. 3. McGraw-Hill, New York, 1972; 2654–2663.

Nyiro, G. and Jablonsky, A. Einige Daten zur Prognose der Epilepsie mit besonderer Berücksichtigung der Konstitution. *Zentralblatt für die gesamte Neurologie und Psychiatrie* 1930; 54:688–689.

Ojemann, L.M., Friel, P., Trejo, W.J., Dudley, D.L. Effect of doxepin on seizure frequency in depressed epileptic patients. *Neurology* 1983; 33:646–648.

O'Keefe, J., Nadel, L. *The Hippocampus as a Cognitive Map*. Oxford University Press, Oxford, 1978.

Olds, J., Milner, P. Positive reinforcement produced by electrical stimulation of septal area and other regions of rat brain. *Journal of Comparative and Physiological Psychology*, 1954; 47:419–427.

Oliver, A.P., Luchins, D.J., Wyatt, R.J. Seizures with neuroleptics. *Archives of General Psychiatry* 1982; 39:206–209.

Onuma, T., Sekine, Y., Komai, S., Akimoto, H. Epileptic psychosis: its electroencephalographic manifestations and follow-up study. *Folia Psychiatrica et Neurologica, Japonica* 1980; 34:337–339.

Onuma, T., Sugai, Y., Yamadera, H., Sekine, Y., Shimazaki, K., Komai, S., Okuma, T., Shimazono, Y. Psychiatric symptoms in patients with epilepsy. In: R. Takahashi, P. Flor-Henry, J. Gruzelier, and S. Niwa, eds. *Cerebral Dynamics, Laterality and Psychopathology*, Elsevier, Holland, 1987; 377–378.

Ottosson, J.O., Experimental studies in the mode of action of ECT. *Acta Psychiatrica Scandinavica* 35:suppl. 1960; 135:1–141.

Ounsted, C., Lindsay The long term outcome of temporal lobe epilepsy in childhood. In: E.H. Reynolds and M.R. Trimble, eds. *Epilepsy and Psychiatry*, Churchill Livingstone, Edinburgh, 1981; 185–215.

Oxbury, J., Adams, C.B.T. Neurosurgery for Epilepsy. *British Journal of Hospital Medicine* 1989; 41:372–377.

Palkanis, A., Drake, M. E., Kuruvilla, J., Blake, K. Forced normalisation. *Archives of Neurology* 1987; 44:289–292.

Papez, J.W. A proposed mechanism of emotion. *Archives of neurology and psychiatry* 1937; 38:725–733.

Parant, V. Des impulsions irrésistibles des épileptiques. *Congress des Médicin alien et neurologie*. Bordeaux 1895; 54.

Parnas, J., Korsgaard, S., Krautwald, O., Jensen, P.S. Chronic psychosis in epilepsy. *Acta Psychiatrica Scandinavica* 1982; 66:282–293.

Penfield, W. Discussion. In: M. Baldwin and P. Bailey, eds. *Temporal lobe epilepsy*, Thomas, Springfield, 1958; 484–485.

Penfield, W., Jasper, H. *Epilepsy and the Functional Anatomy of the Human Brain*. Little, Brown & Co., Boston, 1954.

Penfield, W., Paine, K. Results of surgical therapy for focal epileptic seizures. *Canadian Medical Association Journal* 1955; 73:515–531.

Penfield, W., Perot, P. The brain's record of auditory and visual experience—a final summary and discussion. *Brain* 1963; 86:595–696.

Perez, M. M., Trimble, M. R. Epileptic psychosis—diagnostic comparison with process schizophrenia. *British Journal of Psychiatry* 1980; 137:245–249.

Perez, M. M., Trimble, M. R., Murray, N. M. F., Reider, I. Epileptic psychosis: an evaluation of PSE profiles. *British Journal of Psychiatry* 1985; 146:155–163.

Perucca, L., Manzo, L., Crema, A. Pharmacokinetic interactions between antiepileptic drugs and psychotropic drugs. In: M.R. Trimble, ed. *The Psychopharmacology of Epilepsy* Wiley, Chichester, 1985; 95–105.

Peters, J. G. Dopamine, noradrenalines and serotonin, spinal fluid metabolites in temporal lobe epileptic patients with schizophrenic symptomatology. *European Neurology* 1979; 18:15–18.

Peterson, G.M, McLean, S., Millingen, K.S. Determinants of patient compliance with anticonvulsant drugs. *Epilepsia* 1982; 23:607–614.

Pichot, P. *A Century of Psychiatry.* Roger Da Costa, Paris, 1983.

Pinel, P. A treatise on insanity. Translated by D. D. Davis. W. Todd, Sheffield, 1806.

Pippenger, C.E. Pharmacodynamics of antiepileptic drugs. In: R.M. Post, M.R. Trimble, and C.E. Pippenger, eds. *Clinical Use of Anticonvulsants in Psychiatric Disorders*, Demos, New York, 1989; 89–97.

Polkey, C.E. Effects of anterior temporal lobectomy apart from the relief of seizures. *Journal of the Royal Society of Medicine* 1983; 76:354–358.

Polkey, C.E. Neurosurgery. In: J. Laidlaw, A. Richens, and J. Oxley, eds. *A Textbook of Epilepsy.* Churchill Livingstone, Edinburgh, 1988; 484–510.

Pond, D.A. Psychiatric aspects of epilepsy. *Journal of the Indian Medical Profession* 1957; 3:1441–1451.

Pond, D.A. Epilepsy and personality disorders. In: P.L. Vinken and C.W. Bruyn, eds. *Handbook of Clinical Neurology 15.* North Holland Publishing Co, Amsterdam, 1974.

Pond, D.A., Bidwell, B.A. A survey of epilepsy in fourteen general practices II. Social and psychological aspects. *Epilepsia* 1959; 1:285–299.

Post, R.M. Use of anticonvulsants in the treatment of manic-depressive illness. In: R.M. Post, M.R. Trimble, and C.E. Pippenger, eds. *Clinical Use of Anticonvulsants in Psychiatric Disorders.* Demos, New York, 1989; 113–152.

Post, R.M., Uhde, T.W. Anticonvulsants in non-epileptic psychosis. In: M.R. Trimble and T.G. Bolwig, eds. *Aspects of Epilepsy and Psychiatry.* Wiley, Chichester, 1986; 177–212.

Post, R.M., Putnam, F., Uhde, T.W., Weiss, S.R.B. ECT as an anticonvulsant. In: S. Malitz and H. Sackeim, eds. ECT *Annals of the New York Academy of Sciences*, vol. 462, 1986; 376–388.

Post, R.M., Rubinow, D.R., Uhde, T.W., Ballenger, J.C., and Linnoila, M. Dopaminergic effects of carbamazepine. *Archives of General Psychiatry* 1986; 43:392–396.

Post, R.M., Trimble, M.R., Pippenger, C.E., *Clinical use of Anticonvulsants in Psychiatric Disorders.* Demos, New York, 1989.

Price, J. The efferent projections of the amygdaloid complex in the rat, cat and monkey. In: Y. Ben-Ari, ed. *The Amygdaloid Complex.* Elsevier, North Holland, 1981; 121–132.

Prichard, J.C. *A Treatise on Diseases of the Nervous System.* Thomas & George Underwood, London, 1822.

Pritchard, P.B., Lombroso, C.T., McIntyre, M. Psychological complications of TLE. *Neurology* 1980; 30:227–232.

Procci, W.R. Schizoaffective psychosis: fact or fiction. *Archives of General Psychiatry* 1976; 33:1167–1178.

Racine, R.J. Mechanisms of Kindling. In: T.G. Bolwig and M.R. Trimble, eds. *The Clinical Relevance of Kindling.* Wiley, Chichester, 1989; 15–31.

Radtke, R. A., Hanson, M. W., Coleman, E., Glantz, M. J., Walczak, T. S. Extra temporal PET hypometabolism after temporal lobectomy. *Epilepsia* 1989; 30:666.

Ramani, V., Gumnit, R.J. Intensive monitoring of interictal psychosis in epilepsy. *Annals of Neurology* 1982; 11:613–622.

Ramón y Cajal, S. Studies on the cerebral cortex. Translated by L. M. Kraft. Year Book, Chicago, 1955.

Rasmussen, T.B. Surgical treatment of complex partial seizures. *Epilepsia*, suppl. 1 24: 1983; 565–576.

Rausch, R. Psychological Evaluation. In: J. Engel, ed. *Surgical Treatment of the Epilepsies*, Raven Press, New York, 1987; 181–195.

Rausch, R., Crandall, P.H. Psychological status related to surgical control of temporal lobe seizures. *Epilepsia* 1982; 23:191–202.

Rayport, M., Ferguson, S.M. Qualitative modification of sensory reponses to amygdaloid stimulation in man by interview content and context. *Electroencephalography and Clinical Neurophysiology* 1974; 34:714.

Remick, R.A., Fine, S.H. Antipsychotic drugs and seizures. *Journal of Clinical Psychiatry* 1979; 40:78–80.

Reynolds, E.H. Schizophrenia-like psychoses of epilepsy and disturbances of folate and vitamin B12 metabolism induced by anticonvulsant drugs. *British Journal of Psychiatry* 1967; 113:911–919.

Reynolds, E. H. Mental effects of anticonvulsants and folic acid metabolism. *Brain* 1968; 91:197–204.

Reynolds, E.H. Biological Factors in Epilepsy and Psychiatry. In: E.H. Reynolds and M.R. Trimble, eds. *Epilepsy and Psychiatry*. Churchill Livingstone, Edinburgh 1981; 264–290.

Reynolds, G.P. Increased concentrations and lateral asymmetry of amygdala dopamine in schizophrenia. *Nature* 1983; 305:527–529.

Reynolds, J.R. *Epilepsy*. Churchill, London, 1861.

Rickles, W.H. UCLA conference: clinical neurophysiology. *Annals of Internal Medicine* 1969; 71:619–645.

Riese, W. Ueber den Stilwandel bei Vincent Van Gogh. *Zeitschrift für die gesamte Neurologie und Psychiatrie*, 1925.

Riese, W. *The Conception of Disease*. Philosophical Library, New York, 1953.

Riese, W. *A History of Neurology*. M.D. Publications, New York, 1959.

Roberts, G.W., Done, D.J., Burton, C., Crow, T.J. A "mock up" of schizophrenia: temporal lobe epilepsy and schizophrenia-like psychosis. *Biological Psychiatry—in press*, 1990.

Roberts, G. W., Polak, J. M., Crow, T. J. Peptide circuitry of the limbic system. In: M. R. Trimble and E. Zarifian, eds. *Psychopharmacology of the limbic system*. Oxford University Press, Oxford, 1984; 226–243.

Roberts, J.K.A. *Differential Diagnosis in Neuropsychiatry*. Wiley, Chichester, 1984.

Robertson, M.M., Trimble, M.R. Depressive illness in patients with epilepsy: a review. *Epilepsia* suppl. 2, 1983; 24:109–116.

Robertson, M.M., Trimble, M.R., Townsend, H.R.A. The phenomenology of depression in epilepsy. *Epilepsia*, 1987; 28:364–372.

Rodin, E.A., Dejong, R.N., Waggoner, R.W., Bagchi, B.K. Relationship between certain forms of psychomotor epilepsy and schizophrenia. *Archives of Neurology and Psychiatry*, 1957; 77:449–463.

Rodin, E., Katz, M., Lennox, D. Differences between patients with temporal lobe seizures and those with other forms of epileptic attacks. *Epilepsia*, 1976; 17:313–320.

Rodin, E., Schmaltz, S. The Bear-Fedio Personality Inventory. *Neurology*, 1984; 34:591–596.

Rodin, E. Schmaltz, S., Twitty, G. What does the Bear-Fedio Inventory measure? In: R.J. Porter, R.H. Mattson, A.A. Ward Jr., and M. Dam, eds. The XVth *Epilepsy International Symposium*. Raven Press, New York, 1984; 551–555.

Roger, J., Grangeon, H., Guey, J., Lob, H. Incidences psychiatriques et psychologiques du traitment par l'éthosuccimide chez les épileptiques. *L'encephale*, 1968; 57:407–438.

Roskill, M. *The letters of Vincent Van Gogh*. Atheneum, New York, 1986.

Rosvold, H.E., Mirsky, A.F., Pribram, K.H. Influence of amygdalectomy on social behaviour in monkeys. *Journal of Comparative and Psychological Psychology*, 1954; 47:173–180.

Routtenberg, A. Participation of brain stimulation reward substrates in memory: anatomical and biochemical evidence. *Federation Proceedings* 1979; 38:2446–2453.

Rudorfer, M.V., Risby, M.D., Hsiao, J.K., Linnoila, M., Potter, W.Z. ECT alters monoamines in a different manner from that of antidepressant drugs. *Psychopharmacology Bulletin* 1988; 24:396–399.

Sackeim, H.A., Decina, P., Portnoy, S., Neeley, P., Malitz, S. Studies of dosage, seizure threshold and seizure duration in ECT. *Biological Psychiatry* 1987; 22:249–268.

Samt, P. Epileptische Irreseinsformen. *Archive für Psychiatrie und Nervenkrankheiten* 1875, 1876; 5:393–444; 6:110–216.

Sander, J. W., Hart, Y. M., Trimble, M. R. Shorvon, S. D. Vigabatrin and psychosis. *Journal of Neurology, Neurosurgery and Psychiatry* 1991 (*in press*).

Savage, G. Epilepsy and Insanity. In: D.H. Tuke, eds *A Dictionary of Psychological Medicine*, vol. 1, Churchill, London, 1892; 452–454.

Savard, G., Andermann, F., Remillard, G.M., Oliver, A. Postical psychosis following partial complex seizures is analogous to Todd's paralyses. In: P. Wolf, M. Dam, D. Janz, and F.E. Dreifuss, eds. *Advances in Epileptology*, vol. 16, Raven Press, New York, 1987; 603–660.

Sawyer, C.H. Triggering of the pituitary by the CNS. In: P. Bullock, ed. *Physiological Triggers*. Waverly Press, Baltimore, 1957; 164–174.

Scheibel A.B. Are complex Partial Seizures a sequela of Temporal lobe dysgenesis. In: D. Smith, D.

Treiman, M.R. Trimble, eds. *Neurobehaviour Problems in Epilepsy*. Raven Press, New York, 1991; 59–75.

Scheibel, M.E., Crandall, P.H., Scheibel, A.B. The hippocampal dentate complex in temporal lobe epilespy. *Epilepsia* 1974; 15:55–80.

Schmitz, B., Wolf, P. Psychosis in epilepsy: frequency and relation to different types of epilepsy. Presented at the World Congress of Epilepsy, New Delhi, India, October, 1989.

Schneider, K. Primary and secondary symptoms in schizoprenia. In S.R. Hirsch and M. Shepherd, eds. *Themes and Variations in European Psychiatry* John Wright, Bristol (1974), 1957; 40–46.

Schneider, K. *Clinical Psychopathology*, translated by M.W. Hamilton and E.W. Anderson. Grune and Stratton, New York, 1959.

Schreiner, L., Kling, A. Rhinencephalon and behaviour, *American Journal of Physiology* 1956; 184:486–490.

Schwartz, M.S., Scott, D.F. Isolated petit mal status presenting *de novo* in middle age. *Lancet* 1971; 2:1399–1401.

Sem-Jacobsen, C. W., Peterson, M. C., Lazarte, J. A., Dodge, H. W., Holman, C. B. Intracerebral electrographic recordings from psychotic patients during hallucinations and agitation. *American Journal of Psychiatry* 1956; 112:278–288.

Sengoku, A., Yagi, K., Seino, M., Wada, T. Risks of occurrence of psychoses in relation to the types of epilepsies and epileptic seizures. *Folia Psychiatrica et Neurologica Japonica* 1983; 37:221–225.

Serafetinides, E.A., Falconer, M.A. The effects of temporal lobectomy in epileptic patients with psychosis. *Journal of Mental Science* 1962; 108:584–593.

Sherwin, I. Clinical and EEG aspects of temporal lobe epilepsy with behaviour disorder, the role of cerebral dominance. *McLean Hospital Journal*, special issue, June, 1977; 40–50.

Sherwin, I. Psychosis associated with epilepsy significance of laterality of the epileptogenic lesion. *Journal of Neurology, Neurosurgery and Psychiatry* 1981; 44:83–85.

Sherwin, I., Peron-Magnan, P., Bancaud, J., Boris, A., Talairach, J. Prevalance of psychosis in epilepsy as a function of the laterality of the epileptogenic lesion. *Archives of Neurology* 1982; 39:621–625.

Shukla, G.D., Srivastava, O.N., Katiyar, B.C., Joshi, V., Mohan, P.K. Psychiatric manifestations in TLE: a controlled study. *British Journal of Psychiatry* 1979; 135:411–417.

Siegel, A., Edinger, H., Dotto, M. Effects of electrical stimulation of the lateral aspects of pre-frontal cortex upon attack behaviour in cats. *Brain* 1975; 93:473–484.

Siegel, R. E. *Gylen on psychology, psychopathology, and function and diseases of the nervous system*. Karger, Basel, 1973.

Sieveking, E.H. *On Epilepsy and Epileptiform Seizures*. Churchill, London, 1861.

Silverstein M.L., Harrow M. First rank symptoms in Post-acute Schizophrenia. *American Journal of Psychiatry* 1978; 135:1481–1486.

Simmel, M.L., Counts, S. Clinical and Psychological results of anterior temporal lobectomy in patients with psychomotor epilepsy. In: M. Baldwin and P. Bailey, eds. *Temporal lobe epilepsy* Charles, C. Thomas. Springfield, 1958; 530–550.

Simon, B. *Mind and Madness in Ancient Greece*. Cornell University Press, Ithaca, 1978.

Slater, E., Beard, A.W. The schizophrenia-like psychoses of epilepsy. *British Journal of Psychiatry* 1963; 109:95–150.

Slater, E., Beard, A.W. The schizophrenia-like psychoses of epilepsy v. Discussion and conclusions. *British Journal of Psychiatry* 1963; 109:143–150.

Slater, E., Glitheroe, E. The schizophrenia-like psychoses of epilepsy iii. Genetical aspects. *British Journal of Psychiatry* 1963; 109:130–133.

Slater, E., Moran, P.A.P. The schizophrenia-like psychoses of epilepsy. Relation between ages of onset. *British Journal of Psychiatry* 1969; 115:599–600.

Small, J.G., Milstein, V., Stevens, J.R. Are psychomotor epileptics different? *Archives of Neurology* 1962; 7:330–338.

Small, J.G., Small, I.F. A controlled study of mental disorders associated with epilepsy. *Recent advances in Biological Psychiatry* 1967; 9:171–181.

Small, J.G., Small, I.F., Hayden, M.P. Further psychiatric investigations of patients with temporal and non-temporal lobe epilepsy. *American Journal of Psychiatry* 1966; 123:303–310.

Sommer, W. Erkrankung des Ammonshorns als aetiologisches Moment der Epilepsie. *Archives für Psychiatrie* 1880; 10:631–675.

Sorensen, A.S., Hansen, H., Hogenhaven, H., Bolwig, T.G. Ego function in epilepsy. *Acta Psychiatrica Scandinavica* 1988; 78:211–221.

Spratling, W.P. *Epilepsy and its treatment*. Saunders, Philadelphia, 1904.

Standage, K. Schizophreniform psychosis among epileptics in a mental hospital. *British Journal of Psychiatry* 1973; 123:231–232.

Standage, K.F., Fenton, G.W. Psychiatric symptom profiles of patients with epilepsy: a controlled investigation. *Psychological Medicine* 1975; 5:152–160.

Stark-Adamec, C., Adamec, R.E., Graham, J.M., Hicks, R.C., Bruun-Meyer, S.E. Complexities in the complex partial seizures personality controversy. *Psychiatric Journal of the University of Ottowa* 1985; 10:231–236.

Stephan, H. Allocortex. In: W. Bargmann, ed. *Handbuch der mikroskopischen Anatomie der Menschen,* Springer, Berlin, 1975.

Stevens, J.R. Psychiatric implications of psychomotor epilepsy. *Archives of General Psychiatry* 1966; 14:461–471.

Stevens, J.R. Biologic background of psychosis in epilepsy. In: F. Canger, F. Angeleri, and J.K. Penry, eds. *Advances in Epileptology: XIth International Epilepsy Symposium,* New York, Raven Press, 1980; 167–172.

Stevens, J.R. Neuropathology of schizophrenia. *Archives of General Psychiatry* 1982; 29:177–189.

Stevens, J. All that spikes is not fits. In: M.R. Trimble and E.H. Reynolds, eds. *What is Epilepsy,* Churchill, Edinburgh, 1986; 97–115.

Stevens, J.R. Epilepsy and psychosis: neuropathological studies of six cases. In: M.R. Trimble and T.W. Bolwig, eds. *Aspects of Epilepsy and Psychiatry,* Wiley, Chichester, 1986; pp. 117–145.

Stevens, J.R. Epilepsy, psychosis and schizophrenia. *Schizophrenia Research* 1988; 1:79–89.

Stevens, J.R. Post operative psychosis. Manuscript in preparation, 1991.

Stevens, J.R., Hermann, B. Temporal lobe epilepsy, psychopathology and violence: the state of the evidence. *Neurology* 1981; 31:1127–1132.

Stevens, J.R., Livermore, A. Kindling in mesolimbic dopamine system. *Neurology* 1978; 28:36–46.

Stevens, J.R., Livermore, A. Telemetered EEG in schizophrenia: spectral analysis during abnormal behaviour episodes. *Journal of Neurology, Neurosurgery and Psychiatry* 1982; 45:385–395.

Stevens, J.R., Milstein, V., Goldstein, S. Psychometric test performance in relation to the psychopathology of epilepsy. *Archives of General Psychiatry* 1972; 26:532–538.

Stransky, E. Zur Lehre der kombinierten Psychosen. *Allgemaine Zeitschrift für Psychiatrie* 1906; 63:73–94.

Suddath, R.L., Casanova, M.F., Goldberg, T.E., Daniel, D.G., Kelsoe, J.R., Weinberger, D.R. Temporal lobe pathology in schizophrenia: a quantitative MRI study. *American Journal of Psychiatry* 1989; 146:464–472.

Sydenham, T. *The Whole Works,* 11th edition, translated by J. Peechey. Ware, London, 1740.

Symonds, C. Discussion. *Proceedings of the Royal Society of Medicine* 1962; 55:4–5.

Taylor, D.C. Ontogenesis of chronic epileptic psychoses: A re-analysis. *Psychological Medicine* 1971; 1:247–253.

Taylor, D.C. Mental state and temporal lobe epilepsy. *Epilepsia* 1972; 13:727–765.

Taylor, D.C. Factors influencing the occurrence of schizophrenia-like psychosis in patients with temporal lobe epilepsy. *Psychological Medicine* 1975; 5:249–254.

Taylor, D.C. Epileptic experience, schizophrenia, and the temporal lobe. *McLean Hospital Journal, special issue,* 1977; 22–39.

Taylor, D. C. Brain lesions, surgery, seizures and mental symptoms In: E. H. Reynolds and M. R. Trimble, eds. *Epilepsy and psychiatry.* Churchill Livingstone, Edinburgh, 1981; 227–241.

Taylor, D.C., Falconer, M.A. Clinical, socio-economic and psychological changes after temporal lobectomy for epilepsy. *British Journal of Psychiatry* 1968; 114:1247–1261.

Taylor, D.C., Lochery, M. Temporal lobe epilepsy: origin and significance of simple and complex auras. *Journal of Neurology, Neurosurgery and Psychiatry* 1987; 50:673–681.

Taylor, D.C., Marsh, S.M. Implications of long-term–follow-up in epilepsy: with a note on the cause of death. *Epilepsy: The 8th International Symposium,* J.K. Penry, ed. Raven Press, New York, 1977; 27–34.

Taylor, D.C., Marsh, S.M. Hughlings Jackson's Dr. Z: The paradigm of temporal lobe epilepsy. *Journal of Neurology, Neurosurgery and Psychiatry* 1980; 43:758–767.

Taylor, J. *Selected Writings of John Hughlings Jackson,* vol. 2. Staples Press, London, 1958.

Taylor, M.A., Fleminger, J.J. ECT for schizophrenia, *Lancet* 1980; 1:1380–1383.

Tellenbach, H. Epilepsie als Anfallsleiden und als Psychose. *Der Nervenarzt* 1965; 36:190–202.

Temkin, O. *The falling sickness.* Johns Hopkins University Press, Baltimore, 1971.

Terzian, H. Observations on the clinical symptomatology of bilateral partial or total removal of the temporal lobes in man. In: M. Baldwin and P. Bailey, eds. *Temporal Lobe Epilepsy.* Thomas, Springfield, 1958; 510–529.

Thompson, P.J., Trimble, M.R. Anticonvulsant drugs and cognitive function. *Epilepsia* 1982; 23:531–544.

Tissot, S.A. Traité de l'épilepsie. Paris, 1770.

Tissot, S.A. L'onanism, dissertation sur les maladies produites par la masturbation, 9th edition. Lausanne, 1782.

Tizard, B. The personality of epileptics: a discussion of the evidence. *Psychological Bulletin* 1962; 59:196–210.

Todd, R.B. Clinical lectures on paralysis, certain diseases of the brain and other affections of the nervous system. London, 1856.

Toone, B.K. Psychoses of epilepsy. In: E.H. Reynolds and M.R. Trimble, eds. *Epilepsy and Psychiatry*. Churchill Livingstone, Edinburgh, 1981; 113–137.

Toone, B.K., Fenton, G.W. Epileptic seizures induced by psychotropic drugs. *Psychological Medicine* 1977; 7:265–270.

Toone, B.K., Dawson, J., Driver, M.V. Psychoses of epilepsy: a radiological evaluation. *British Journal of Psychiatry* 1982; 140:244–248.

Toone, B.K., Garralda, M.E., Ron, M.A. The psychoses of epilepsy and the functional psychoses: a clinical and phenomenological comparison. *British Journal of Psychiatry* 1982; 141:256–261.

Trimble, M.R. The relationship between epilepsy and schizophrenia: a biochemical hypothesis. *Biological Psychiatry* 1977; 12:299–304.

Trimble, M.R. Non-MAOI antidepressants and epilepsy: a review. *Epilepsia* 1978; 19:241–250.

Trimble, M.R. Serum prolactin in epilepsy and hysteria. *British Medical Journal* 1978; 2:1682.

Trimble, M.R. Hysteria. In: E.H. Reynolds and M.R. Trimble, eds. *The Bridge between Neurology and Psychiatry*. Churchill Livingstone, Edinburgh, 1989; 159–176.

Trimble, M.R. *Neuropsychiatry*, Wiley, Chichester, 1981.

Trimble, M.R. Functional disorders. *British Medical Journal* 1982; 285:1768–1770.

Trimble, M.R. Hypergraphia. In: M.R. Trimble and T.G. Bolwig, eds. *Aspects of Epilepsy and Psychiatry*. Wiley, Chichester, 1986; 75–88.

Trimble, M.R. Positive and negative symptoms in psychiatry. *British Journal of Psychiatry* 1986; 148:587–589.

Trimble M.R. *Biological Psychiatry*. Wiley, Chichester, 1988.

Trimble, M.R. Hysteria. In: E.H. Reynolds and M.R. Trimble, eds. *The Bridge between Neurology and Psychology*. Churchill Livingstone, Edinborough, 1989; 159–176.

Trimble, M.R., Perez, M.M. Quantification of psychopathology in adult patients with epilepsy. In: B.M. Kulig, H. Meinardi, and G. Stores, eds. *Epilepsy and Behaviour 1979* Lisse. Swets and Zeitlinger, 1980; 118–126.

Trimble, M.R., Perez, M.M. The phenomenology of the chronic psychoses of epilepsy. In: W.P. Koella and M.R. Trimble, eds. *Temporal Lobe Epilepsy, Mania and Schizophrenia and the Limbic System*. Karger, Basel, 1982; 98–105.

Tucker, D.M., Novelly, R.A., Walker, P.J. Hyperreligiosity in temporal lobe epilepsy: re-defining the relationship. *Journal of Nervous and Mental Disease* 1987; 115:181–184.

Turner, A. *Epilepsy*. Macmillan, London, 1907.

Turner, W.A. *Three Lectures on Epilepsy*. J. MacKenzie, Edinburgh, 1910.

Ungerstedt, U. Stereotaxic mapping of the monoamine pathways in the rat brain. *Acta Physiologica Scandinavica* 1971; 197: suppl. 367:1–48.

Van Hoesen, G.U. The parahippocampal gyrus. *Trends in Neurosciences* 1982; 5:345–349.

Vetulani, J., Lebrecht, U., Pilc, A. Enhancement of responsiveness of the central serotonergic system and serotonin-2 receptor density in rat frontal cortex by ECT. *European Journal of Pharmacology* 1981; 76:81–85.

Walker, E.A., Blumer, D. Behaviour effects of temporal lobectomy. In: D. Blumer, ed. *Psychiatric Aspects of Epilepsy*. American Psychiatric Press. 1984; 295–323.

Waxman, S.G., Geschwind, N. The interictal behaviour syndromes of temporal lobe epilepsy. *Archives of General Psychiatry* 1975 32:1580–1586.

Wells, C.E. Transient ictal psychosis. *Archives of General Psychiatry* 1975; 32:1201–1203.

White, L.E. Development and morphology of human nucleus accumbens. In: R.B. Chronister and J.F. De France, eds. *The Neurobiology of the Nucleus Accumbens* Haer Institute, New Jersey, 1981; 198–209.

White, S., Besag, F., Fenwick, P., Pelosi, A. CT attenuation densities in patients with epilepsy and psychiatric disorder (unpublished manuscript).

Whitman, S., Hermann, B.P., Gordon, A. Psychopathology in epilepsy: how great the risk. *Biological Psychiatry* 1984; 19:213–236.

W.H.O. *Report of the International Pilot Study of Schizophrenia.* W.H.O., Geneva, 1963.

Wiesel, F.A., Wik, G., Sjogren, I., Blomquist, G., Grettz, T., Stone-Elander, S. Regional brain glucose metabolism in drug free schizophrenia patients and clinical correlates. *Acta Psychiatrica Scandinavica* 1987; 76:628–641.

Wieser, H.G. Depth recorded limbic seizures and psychopathology. *Neuroscience and Behaviour Reviews* 1983; 7:427–440.

Wieser, H.G. Selective amygdalo-hippocampectomy for temporal lobe epilepsy. *Epilepsia* 1988; suppl. 2, 29:100–113.

Wieser, H.G., Hailemariam, S., Regard, M., Landis, T. Unilateral limbic epileptic status activity: stereo EEG, behavioural, and cognitive data. *Epilepsia* 1985; 26:19–29.

Williams, D. The structure of emotions reflected in epileptic experience. *Brain* 1956; 19:29–67.

Willis, T. *Pathologiae cerebri et nervosi generis specimen*, translated 1681 by S. Pordage. Dring, London, 1667.

Wilmore, L.J., Heilman, K.M., Fennell, E. The effect of chronic seizures on religiosity. *Transactions of the American Neurology Association* 1980; 105:85–87.

Wing, J.K., Cooper, J.E., Sartorius, N. *The Measurement and Classification of Psychiatric Symptoms.* Cambridge University Press, London, 1974.

Wolf, P. Forced Normalisation. In: M.R. Trimble and T.G. Bolwig, eds. *Aspects of Epilepsy and Psychiatry* Wiley, Chichester, 1988; 101–115.

Wolf, P. Acute behavioural symptomatology at disappearance of epileptiform EEG abnormality: paradoxical or "forced" normalisation. In: D. Smith, D. Treiman, and M.R. Trimble, eds. *Neurobehavioral Problems in Epilepsy*, Raven Press, New York, 1991.

Wolf, P., Trimble, M.R. Biological antagonism and epileptic psychosis. *British Journal of Psychiatry* 1985; 146:272–276.

Wrysch, J. Über Schizophrenie bei Epileptikern. *Schweizer Archiv für Neurologie und Psychiatrie* 1933; 31:113–132.

Yakovlev, P. Motility, behaviour and the brain. *Journal of Nervous and Mental Disease* 1948; 107:313–335.

Yde, A. On the relation between schizophrenia, epilepsy and induced convulsions. *Acta Psychiatrica Scandinavica* 1941; 16:325–388.

Ziehen, T. *Psychiatrie*, Leipzig, 1902.

Zielinski, J.J. *Epidemiology and Medical-social Problems of Epilepsy in Warsaw.* Warsaw Psychoneurological Institute, 1974.

Zilboorg, G. *A History of Medical Psychology.* W.W. Norton, New York, 1941.

Subject Index